Withholding and Withdrawing Life-prolonging Medical Treatment

Guidance for decision making

Second edition
incorporating guidance on the Human Rights Act

British Medical Association

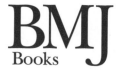

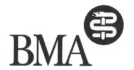

© BMJ Books 2001
BMJ Books is an imprint of the BMJ Publishing Group

First published in 1999
by BMJ Books, BMA House, Tavistock Square,
London WC1H 9JR
First edition 1999
Second edition 2001

www.bmjbooks.com

British Library Cataloguing in Publication Data

A catalogue record for this book is available from the British Library

ISBN 0-7279-1615-7

Typeset by FiSH Books, London
Printed and bound by MPG Books Ltd, Bodmin, Cornwall

Contents

Foreword

Decisions to withhold or withdraw life-prolonging treatment are among the most difficult for patients and health professionals to make. Most people accept that treatment should not be prolonged indefinitely, when it has ceased to provide a benefit for the patient. But doctors, patients and their families, members of the clinical team and society need reassurance that each individual decision is carefully thought through, is based on the best quality information available and follows a widely agreed procedure. This is especially the case in view of the implementation of the Human Rights Act. The guiding principle underlying any decision of this kind must be to protect the dignity, comfort and rights of the patient; to take into account the wishes – if known – of the patient and, where the patient is not competent, the views of those close to the patient. The need for guidance in this area became clear from a wide-ranging consultation exercise, undertaken by the British Medical Association (BMA) in 1998, which also confirmed that one of the most difficult decisions relates to withholding or withdrawing artificial nutrition and hydration.

Confusion has arisen from the fact that guidance from the courts on withdrawing artificial nutrition and hydration specifically refers to patients in persistent vegetative state, without making reference to other serious conditions in which a decision to withhold or withdraw artificial nutrition and hydration might arise. With some conditions, such as advanced dementia or very severe stroke, a practice has developed where, in some cases, a decision is made that life-prolonging treatment, including artificial nutrition and hydration, is not a benefit to the patient and should not be provided or continued. The BMA does not believe that these cases should routinely be subject to court review but considers that there should be in place standard policies and guidance outlining the criteria and steps to be followed in reaching these decisions in all cases. As with all conditions, patients should be assured of uniformly high-quality assessment of their condition and of the potential treatment options available. Guidelines help to ensure that proper and transparent procedures are followed.

This guidance attempts to document the type of factors which should be taken into account, the process which should be followed and the safeguards which should be in place to ensure that these decisions, and decisions to withhold or withdraw other life-prolonging treatments, are made appropriately.

DR MICHAEL WILKS
Chairman, BMA Medical Ethics Committee

Medical Ethics Committee

A publication from the BMA's Medical Ethics Committee (MEC) whose membership for 1998/99 was:

Sir Dilwyn Williams	President, BMA
Professor Brian Hopkinson	Chairman of the Representative Body, BMA
Dr Ian Bogle	Chairman of Council, BMA
Dr W James Appleyard	Treasurer, BMA
Dr Michael Wilks*	Chairman, Medical Ethics Committee
Dr Paddy Glackin	Deputy Chairman, Medical Ethics Committee
Professor Alastair Campbell	Professor of Ethics in Medicine, Bristol
Dr Andrew Carney*	Consultant Psychiatrist, London
Dr Peter Dangerfield	Medical Academic, Liverpool
Professor Robin Downie	Professor of Moral Philosophy, Glasgow
Professor Len Doyal*	Senior Lecturer in Medical Ethics, London
Dr Sam Everington	General Practitioner, London
Mrs Elizabeth Fradd	Nursing Directorate, NHS Executive
Professor Raanan Gillon*	General Practitioner and Professor of Medical Ethics, London
Dr R John Givans	General Practitioner, Yorkshire
Professor J Stuart Horner	Academic, Former Public Health Physician, Preston
Mrs Anne MacLean	Moral Philosopher, Swansea
Professor Sheila McLean*	Director of Institute of Law and Ethics, Glasgow

* Member of the MEC Working Group which considered the responses to the BMA's consultation exercise and prepared the guidance.

Mr Derek Morgan*	Reader in Health Care Law and Jurisprudence, Cardiff
Dr Jane Richards*	Former General Practitioner
Dr Ewen Sim	Histopathologist, Bolton
Dr Jeremy Wight*	Public Health Physician, Sheffield
Sir Cyril Chantler	General Medical Council Observer
Ms Jane O'Brien	General Medical Council Observer
Ms Rosie Wilkinson*	Royal College of Nursing Observer

* Member of the MEC Working Group which considered the responses to the BMA's consultation exercise and prepared the guidance.

Editorial Board

Acknowledgements

The BMA is most grateful to everyone who responded to its consultation exercise carried out during 1998. Over 2,000 responses were received and these were instrumental in deciding the scope and contents of the guidance. Thanks are also due to the many people who gave so generously of their time in commenting on earlier drafts and discussing the very difficult medical, legal and ethical issues with us. Whilst these contributions helped to inform the BMA's views, it should not be assumed that this guidance necessarily reflects the views of all those who contributed. Particular thanks are due to Dr Keith Andrews for providing factual information and advice and for allowing BMA staff to visit the Hospital for Neuro-disability in Putney to discuss the practical dilemmas which arise with him and his staff. We would also like to thank: Dr Timothy Chambers, Ms Sarah Elliston, Ms Marie Fox, Ms Fiona Hass, Mr Michael Hinchliffe, Dr Damian Jenkinson, Professor Bryan Jennett, Mr Simon John, Ms Claire Johnston, Dr John Keown, Dr Vic Larcher, Professor John Lennard-Jones, Dr Simon Lovestone, Professor Michael Lye, Dr Steven Luttrell, Professor John Stanley, Ms Cheryl Viney, Dr Stephen Webster and The UK Acquired Brain Injury Forum. The Medical Ethics Committee is also grateful for the help and advice provided by the BMA's Science and Research Adviser, Dr Bill O'Neill.

Introduction

In medicine, decisions are made on a daily basis about the provision, withholding or withdrawing of treatments, many of which could prolong life. Treatments which could provide a therapeutic benefit are not inevitably given but are weighed according to a number of factors, such as the patient's wishes, the treatment's invasiveness, side effects, limits of efficacy and the resources available. In relation to many conditions, a body of accepted practice has been building about the criteria for treatment and non-treatment decisions. Nevertheless, the BMA is concerned that comprehensive guidance outlining the criteria and steps to be followed in making these decisions, particularly where the decision involves assessing the best interests of incompetent patients, does not exist. This is due partly to the fact that many of the techniques for prolonging the biological functions of severely brain-damaged people are relatively new. The main disadvantage of not having clear written policies and guidance is that patients may suffer by being subjected to inappropriate treatments or by having treatment withdrawn when it could provide a benefit. Without clear guidance, the public may feel that different standards are being applied in similar cases and doctors do not necessarily have any benchmark by which to audit their own decisions. Where published guidance on some aspects of this subject exists, this document takes account of it.[1] In this document, the BMA seeks to provide a coherent and comprehensive set of principles which apply to all decisions to withhold or withdraw life-prolonging treatment. It is hoped that this general guidance will stimulate the development of local policies and guidelines as part of a wider network of safeguards for doctors and patients.

Though the publication of the first edition of this guidance preceded implementation of the Human Rights Act 1998 on 2 October 2000, that piece of legislation is clearly relevant to these types of decisions. Indeed, this second edition of the guidance has been substantially revised to take the Act into account. (The BMA has also prepared general guidance on the impact of the Human Rights Act on medical decision making.) Under the terms of the Act all public authorities have to act in accordance with the bulk of the rights set out in the European Convention on Human Rights, and all statutes have to be interpreted so far as possible to be in accordance with those rights. The Convention rights include: the right to life (Article 2); the right not to be tortured or subjected to inhuman or degrading treatment (Article 3); the right to security of the person (Article 5); the right to respect for privacy (Article 8); the right to freedom of thought, conscience and religion (Article 9); the right to freedom of expression including the right to receive and impart information (Article 10); and the right not to be discriminated against in the enjoyment of these various rights (Article 14). No legislation so pervasive as the Human Rights Act has ever been passed by a British legislature, and its impact on UK law is likely to be dramatic. However the basic principles that underpin the Act – most significantly respect for human dignity and respect for legality – are already ideas that underpin much of the ethical and legal framework within which current practice in the withholding and withdrawing of life-prolonging treatment occurs. The requirements of the Human Rights Act reflect, very closely, existing good medical practice. So the Act is less foreign in this field than it will be in other areas of the law. However it speaks a new legal language and this does need to be taken into account. It also extends its duties directly only to public authorities, without defining what these are. In this guidance we have not tried to answer this question, but have rather made an assumption that all health professionals and health teams, howsoever constituted, should regard themselves as bound by the terms of the Act.

Few issues in medicine are more complex and difficult than those addressed by patients, their relatives and their doctors concerning the decision to withhold or withdraw life-prolonging treatment. Technological developments continually extend the range of treatment options available to prolong life when organ or system failure would naturally result in death. Cardiopulmonary resuscitation, renal dialysis, artificial nutrition, hydration and ventilation prolong life and, in some cases, allow time for natural recovery to occur but these techniques in themselves cannot reverse a patient's disease. Patients with progressive conditions such as Alzheimer's disease or Motor Neurone Disease can have their lives prolonged considerably by the application of technology, yet their irreversibly deteriorating conditions will eventually result in death. The condition of other patients, for example those with very severe brain damage, may remain stable for many years if life-prolonging treatment is provided but with no hope of recovering more than very minimal levels of awareness of their surroundings. They may lack ability to interact with others or capacity for self-directed action. In such severely damaged patients, treatment to prolong life by artificial means may fail to provide sufficient benefit to justify the intervention and the proper course of action may be to withhold or withdraw further treatment.

Health professionals are well aware that the availability of a technique does not necessarily mean that its use would be appropriate in every case. It is evident, however, that the lack of guidance about the type of circumstances in which non-treatment decisions would be appropriate, and the factors which should be taken into account in reaching these decisions, has led to considerable confusion and concern. This anxiety is found among health professionals, who are worried about the scope of their discretion for making such decisions, and among patients and their relatives who are worried that treatment may either be withdrawn prematurely or continued long past the stage at which it continues to be a benefit.

Matters of life and death give rise to emotive and impassioned debate. Such responses cannot and should not be ignored. The symbolic importance of appearing to "give up" on some patients cannot be over-estimated and sensitivity is required to ensure that such impressions are not given. As we stress throughout, good communications, listening to all relevant parties and thoroughly investigating the options are central to good decision making. The decisions addressed in this document may generate conflicting views. This guidance urges a cautious and thoughtful approach to such decisions, recognising the difficult areas of ethical tension, the legal uncertainties[2] and the possibility of divergence of medical opinion, whilst attempting to provide practical assistance to those patients and health professionals who must confront these issues.

PART 1   Setting the scene for decision making

1.   The primary goal of medicine

1.1   The primary goal of medical treatment is to benefit the patient by restoring or maintaining the patient's health as far as possible, maximising benefit and minimising harm. If treatment fails, or ceases, to give a net benefit to the patient (or if the patient has competently refused the treatment) that goal cannot be realised and the justification for providing the treatment is removed. Unless some other justification can be demonstrated, treatment that does not provide net benefit to the patient may, ethically and legally, be withheld or withdrawn and the goal of medicine should shift to the palliation of symptoms.

Treatment which achieves its physiological aim may fail to provide a net benefit to the patient because it is unable to achieve a level of recovery which justifies the corresponding burdens of the treatment. Or, the treatment may keep the patient alive but be unable to stop the progression of the disease or provide any hope of the patient recovering self-awareness, awareness of others and the ability intentionally to interact with them. Whilst the BMA reiterates its opposition to active, intentional measures taken with the purpose of ending a patient's life, it does not hold to the view that there is an absolute value in being alive regardless of the patient's wishes or medical condition.

Debate on this subject has tended to focus on assessing the justification for withdrawing or withholding treatment. In the BMA's view the emphasis should shift to considering whether the benefits of the treatment justify the intervention. For every proposed or actual medical intervention, a judgment should be made about whether that intervention would be worthwhile, in the sense of providing some benefit to the individual patient, recognising that each patient has his or her own values, beliefs, wishes and philosophies. In the BMA's opinion, this approach, of considering benefit, reflects both the emphasis on human dignity in the Human Rights Act and the approach adopted by the House of Lords in its consideration of the case of Tony Bland.[3] Bland was in a persistent vegetative state following the Hillsborough Stadium football disaster. When considering whether artificial nutrition and hydration could be withdrawn, Lord Goff of Chieveley said the correct question was not whether it was "in his best interests that the treatment should be ended. But... whether it is in his best interests that treatment which has the effect of artificially prolonging his life should be continued". Considered in this way, a decision to withhold or withdraw treatment is a decision not to provide a treatment which does not confer a net health benefit upon the patient.

1.2   Prolonging a patient's life usually, but not always, provides a health benefit to that patient. It is not an appropriate goal of medicine to prolong life at all costs, with no regard to its quality or the burdens of treatment.

High regard for value of life does not necessarily imply a duty always to give life-prolonging treatment. One of the incorporated European Convention rights in the Human Rights Act is that "[E]veryone's right to life shall be protected by law" (Article 2(1)). This is a positive obligation to preserve life as well as a negative order not to kill, but the positive obligation is not one that should be pushed too far. The Article 2(1) guarantee in no way involves an absolute obligation indefinitely to prolong life at all costs and without regard to the consequences for the patient of such a prolongation (see section 19.1). It is not the case that all lives must be prolonged by artificial means for as long as technically possible. Competent patients sometimes decide that the stage has been reached beyond which, for them, continued treatment aimed at prolonging life, although possible, would be inappropriate. Where patients are not competent, these decisions must be taken in a way which is perceived to reflect their wishes or best interests or, where this is not achievable, which is not contrary to their interests or rights. This may include a decision not to provide or continue to provide an intervention which is not of benefit to the patient even if the withholding or withdrawing of that treatment allows the patient to die earlier than if the treatment were provided or continued.

Terms such as "quality of life" are problematic and ambivalent. They can imply that some people are less valued. But, whether articulated or not, the concept of "quality of life" is unavoidable. It is common currency among patients and their relatives as a way of judging whether they should pursue further medical interventions. A vital part of the treatment decision rests on the issue of whether the proposed measures can restore the patient to a way of living he or she would be likely to consider of reasonable "quality", despite any side effects or disadvantages of treatment. The Human Rights Act's strong emphasis on human dignity is another way of stressing this central ethical principle. It must always be clear that the doctor's role is not to assess the value or worth of the *patient* but that of the *treatment*. If the latter cannot benefit the patient, in terms of restoring that person's health to a level that he or she would find acceptable, its use must be open to question.

The courts have specifically stated that the "quality of life" which could reasonably be expected following treatment is an appropriate factor to take into account when making treatment decisions. The decision to withhold life-prolonging treatment from a patient, R,[4] who was born with a serious malformation of the brain and cerebral palsy, was challenged in the High Court in 1996 on the grounds that it was "irrational and unlawful" to permit medical treatment to be withheld on the basis of an assessment of a patient's quality of life. That appeal was dismissed. Drawing on the 1990 case of *Re J*,[5] which concerned a baby who was born prematurely with severe brain damage, the court decided that it was appropriate to consider whether the patient's life, if treatment was given, would be "so afflicted as to be intolerable". If the patient's condition has reached that level of severity and treatment is unable to lead to any improvement, this is one of the situations in which treatment could, legally and ethically, be withdrawn. The Human Rights Act guarantees protection for life but it also declares that "[N]o one shall be subjected to torture or to inhuman or degrading treatment or punishment" (Article 3). Life should not be artificially preserved where the treatment to secure this leaves a patient in what might be judged as "an inhuman or degrading state". The doctor must balance his or her duty to protect life with his or her obligation not to subject the patient to inhuman or degrading treatment. It is likely that in time case law will clarify how this is to be judged. It may well be that the interpretation of "inhuman or degrading" will follow the courts' previous decisions in which the patient's "quality of life" has been a consideration.

Views differ as to what factors should be considered in deciding whether continued provision of life-prolonging treatment would be a benefit to a patient who is unable to express his or her own wishes. Some people believe that there is intrinsic value in being alive and therefore that prolonging life will always provide a benefit to the patient regardless of any other factors. In this absolute form, this is not a view which the BMA shares. The vast majority of people with, even very severe, physical or mental disabilities are able to experience and gain pleasure from some aspects of their lives. Where, however, the disability is so profound that individuals have no or minimal levels of awareness of their own existence and no hope of recovering awareness, or where they suffer severe untreatable pain or other distress, the question arises as to whether continuing to provide treatment aimed at prolonging that life artificially would provide a benefit to them. An important factor which is often considered in making these decisions is whether the person is thought to be aware of his or her environment or own existence as demonstrated by, for example:

- being able to interact with others;
- being aware of his or her own existence and having an ability to take pleasure in the fact of that existence; and
- having the ability to achieve some purposeful or self-directed action or to achieve some goal of importance to him or herself.

If treatment is unable to recover or maintain any of these abilities, this is likely to indicate that its continued provision will not be a benefit to the patient. If any one of these abilities can be achieved, then life-prolonging treatment may be of benefit and it is important to consider these factors within the context of the individual's own wishes and values, where these are known, in order to assess whether the patient would, or could reasonably be expected to, consider life-prolonging treatment to be beneficial.

1.3   The primary goal of medicine – to benefit the patient's health with minimal harm – should be explained to patients and/or those close to them so that they can understand why treatment is given and why, in some circumstances, a decision to withhold or withdraw further life-prolonging treatment may need to be considered.

When treatment fails or ceases to provide a net benefit to the patient, that primary justification for continuing to provide it no longer exists. Where the patient is competent any decision should involve sensitive and detailed discussion with the patient. Where competence is lacking and, following appropriate consultation with those close to the patient (see section 18.3), a decision has been made to withhold or withdraw a particular treatment, the reasons for this should be carefully explained to those close to the patient so that it is not interpreted as "giving up" on or abandoning the patient. Not only is this consultation the ethical way to proceed, it may also frequently be required as a matter of law under Article 8 of the European Convention which obliges health professionals (as it does all public authorities) to respect a person's private and family life.

2.   Scope of this guidance

2.1   The main focus of this guidance is decisions to withdraw or withhold life-prolonging treatment from patients who are likely to live for weeks, months, or possibly years, if treatment is provided but who, without treatment, will or may die earlier. In some areas mention is also made of treatment decisions for those patients whose imminent death is inevitable.

This guidance focuses on the process through which decisions are made to withdraw or withhold life-prolonging treatment from all types of patient – competent adults, incompetent adults, children and babies. Such decisions are taken on a regular basis, throughout the country, where it is decided, for example, that the burdens of further aggressive chemotherapy or dialysis outweigh the benefits for the particular individual. Similarly, a decision may

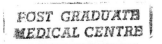

be made that, in the event of cardiac arrest, a patient should not be subjected to cardiopulmonary resuscitation because the chances of recovery, or the level of recovery which could reasonably be expected, would not provide a net benefit to that patient. These decisions are always profound and cannot be taken lightly. The intention of this guidance is to set down what is already established good practice in this area and to suggest some additional safeguards for decisions to withhold or withdraw artificial nutrition and hydration.

3. Definitions

3.1 ***Benefit*: Health professionals have a general duty to provide treatment which benefits their patients. Benefit, in this context, has its ordinary meaning of an advantage or net gain for the patient but is broader than simply whether the treatment achieves a particular physiological goal. It includes both medical and other, less tangible, benefits.**

There are some circumstances where the use of life-prolonging treatment will be justified even though the side effects, burdens and risks of the treatment itself are significant; in other cases the use of such treatment will not be justified. In deciding which treatment should be offered, the expectation must be that the advantages outweigh the drawbacks for the individual patient. Where the patient is competent he or she is the best judge of what represents an acceptable level of burden or risk. Where the patient is not competent, any previously expressed wishes should form a core part of assessing the benefit to that person. To do something to an individual against his or her wishes can, in itself, be a harm to that person and risks also being viewed by the courts as an infringement of their basic rights, in particular those in Article 5, Article 8 and Article 9 of the European Convention. A Jehovah's Witness who has refused a life-prolonging blood transfusion, for example, will, in some sense, be harmed by being given a transfusion against his or her stated wishes. If there is evidence that the individual would not view a particular procedure as offering benefit, that must be taken into account. Judgments should be made according to the strength of evidence available.

The BMA does not consider that the provision of treatment to prolong life will always be a benefit. In the most extreme cases of profound disability, treatment to prolong life artificially may not provide a net benefit to the patient and the goal of medicine should shift to the palliation of symptoms. In such circumstances, the doctors would have done all that they would reasonably be expected to do in discharge of their positive duty to protect life under the Human Rights Act.

3.2 **Life-prolonging treatment: refers to all treatment which has the potential to postpone the patient's death and includes cardiopulmonary resuscitation, artificial ventilation, specialised treatments for particular conditions such as chemotherapy or dialysis, antibiotics when given for a potentially life-threatening infection and artificial nutrition and hydration (see section 3.4).**

Developments in technology mean that patients can increasingly be kept alive when previously their condition would inevitably have resulted in early death. This means that the basic biological functions can be maintained, artificially, in many patients even though there may be no prospect of the patient recovering or developing any awareness of his or her surroundings.

3.3 **Basic care: means those procedures essential to keep an individual comfortable. The administration of medication or the performance of any procedure which is solely or primarily designed to provide comfort to the patient or alleviate that person's pain, symptoms or distress are facets of basic care. This includes warmth, shelter, pain relief, management of distressing symptoms (such as breathlessness or vomiting), hygiene measures (such as the management of incontinence) and the offer of oral nutrition and hydration (see section 3.5).**

Whilst treatment may, in some circumstances, be withheld or withdrawn, appropriate basic care should always be provided unless actively resisted by the patient (if the patient resists, legally, any

7

acceleration of death that occurred would properly be seen as beyond the doctor's control). This does not mean that all facets of basic care must be provided in all cases; a competent patient may be willing to tolerate some pain in order to maintain a level of awareness which permits interaction with relatives and friends. Where, however, the individual is unable to express preferences, procedures which are essential to keep the patient comfortable should be provided. If there is doubt about a patient's comfort, the presumption should be in favour of providing relief from symptoms and distress.

3.4 ***Artificial nutrition and hydration*: refers specifically to those techniques for providing nutrition or hydration which are used to bypass a pathology in the swallowing process. It includes the use of nasogastric tubes, percutaneous endoscopic gastrostomy (PEG feeding) and total parenteral nutrition.[6]**

Following legal judgments, these techniques are classed as medical treatment which may be withdrawn in some circumstances. The BMA believes that withholding or withdrawing artificial nutrition and hydration should be subject to additional safeguards (see Part 3D) including, in some cases, legal review.

Whilst the term "artificial nutrition and hydration" is used in this guidance, it is recognised that neither the nutrition nor the hydration is, in fact, *artificial* although the method for delivering it is. Some people prefer to use terms such as "tube feeding" or "technologically delivered feeding". Since artificial nutrition and hydration has become a widely used and accepted term, however, this terminology has been used throughout this document.

Whether artificial nutrition and hydration constitutes medical treatment or basic care was one of the central questions considered by the House of Lords in the *Bland* case.[7] The view of three of the five Law Lords who considered this case was expressed by Lord Goff as follows:

> *"There is overwhelming evidence that, in the medical profession, artificial feeding is regarded as a form of medical treatment; and even if it is not strictly medical treatment, it must form part of the medical care of the patient."*

This classification of artificial nutrition and hydration as medical treatment, which has been the published view of the BMA since 1992, has been adopted in other subsequent cases in England and Scotland[8] and is now established common law.

The BMA accepts that this is a controversial area where views differ. Some people regard the provision of artificial nutrition and hydration as basic care which should always be provided unless the patient's imminent death is inevitable. Others make a distinction between the insertion of a feeding tube – which is classed as treatment – and the provision of nutrition and hydration through the tube, which is considered basic care.[9] From this perspective decisions not to insert a feeding tube, or not to reinsert it if it becomes dislodged, would be legitimate medical decisions whereas a decision to stop providing nutrition and hydration through an existing tube would not. This distinction was not made by the House of Lords (which specifically rejected any distinction between withholding and withdrawing treatment – see section 6) and is not supported by the BMA. The provision of nutrition and hydration by artificial means requires the use of medical or nursing skills to overcome a pathology in the swallowing mechanism, in the same way that the artificial provision of insulin is given to diabetic patients to overcome the body's own inability to produce that substance.

Whilst classifying artificial nutrition and hydration as treatment, the House of Lords conceded that its withdrawal was a particularly sensitive matter. For the protection of patients and doctors and for the reassurance of the patients' families and the public, it was decided that additional safeguards should be put in place. This was expressed, in the case of patients in a persistent vegetative state, by a recommendation that, in England, Wales and Northern Ireland, each case in which it was proposed to withdraw artificial nutrition and hydration should be subject to review by the court. The Law Commission, in its report on Mental Incapacity,[10] reiterated this need for additional safeguards for the withdrawal of artificial nutrition and hydration but considered that alternatives to a court declaration should be considered.

Confusion has arisen from the fact that the guidance issued by the courts, following the *Bland* judgment, specifically referred to patients in persistent vegetative state without making reference to other serious conditions in which a decision to withhold or withdraw artificial nutrition and hydration might arise. With some conditions, such as advanced dementia or very severe stroke, a practice has developed where, in some cases, a decision is made that life-prolonging treatment, including artificial nutrition and hydration, would not be a benefit to the patient and should not be provided or continued. The BMA does not believe that these cases should routinely be subject to court review but considers that there should be in place standard policies and guidance outlining the criteria and steps to be followed in reaching these decisions. Such guidelines help to ensure that proper and transparent procedures are followed. It is possible that the different approach taken at present to this issue, with patients in a persistent vegetative state being subject to a court review and others not being so subject, is inconsistent with the Human Rights Act guarantee against discrimination in the enjoyment of, among other rights, the right to life guaranteed in Article 2(1). If the courts were to remove the requirement for court review for patients in a persistent vegetative state, as discussed in section 21.4, this could avoid a potential breach of Article 14. The BMA believes that this is an area that needs urgent review in light of the Human Rights Act.

3.5 *Oral nutrition and hydration*: **Where nutrition and hydration are provided by ordinary means – such as by cup, spoon or any other method for delivering food or nutritional supplements into the patient's mouth – or the moistening of a patient's mouth for comfort, this forms part of basic care and should not be withdrawn.**

Food or water to be given by these means should always be offered but should not be forced upon patients who resist or express a clear refusal. It should also not be forced upon patients for whom the process of feeding produces an unacceptable level of burden, such as where it causes unavoidable choking or aspiration of the food or fluid. In the latter case, it would be appropriate to consider whether artificial nutrition and hydration would provide a benefit to the patient, using the guidance set out in Parts 3C and 3D of this document.

Many patients, such as babies, young children and people with disability, may require assistance with feeding but retain the ability to swallow if the food is placed in their mouth; this forms part of basic care. Evidence suggests that when patients are close to death, however, they seldom want nutrition or hydration and its provision may, in fact, exacerbate discomfort and suffering.[11] Good practice should include moistening their mouths as necessary to keep them comfortable.

4. The inevitability of death

4.1 Developments in technology have led to a misperception in society that death can almost always be postponed. There needs to be a recognition that there comes a point in all lives where no more can reasonably or helpfully be done to benefit patients other than keeping them comfortable and free from pain.

With life-prolonging treatment some patients could potentially survive for many years without achieving awareness or being able to interact with others. This has led to unrealistic expectations in society about the extent to which it is possible to postpone death such that death is sometimes seen not as a natural, inevitable event but as a failure of medicine. Societal perceptions need to shift away from the view that life can be prolonged indefinitely back towards a realistic acceptance of the inevitability of death.

5. The inherent uncertainty in medical treatment

5.1 Despite being evidence based, some aspects of medical treatment will always remain uncertain. Death is a certainty for everyone but, except in a small number of cases, diagnosis and prognosis are based on probability and past evidence rather than absolute certainty.

Much fear is engendered by reports of mistaken diagnosis or a belief that had treatment been provided, the patient may have recovered to a level that would have been acceptable to that individual. One of the difficulties for health professionals is that it

11

is often not possible to predict with certainty how any individual will respond to a particular treatment or, in the final stages of an illness, how long the dying process will take. Health professionals have an ethical obligation to keep their skills up to date and to keep abreast of new developments in their specialty and to base their decisions on a reasonable assessment of the facts available. There will, however, always remain some areas of uncertainty and empirical judgments are necessarily based on probabilities rather than certainties. Wider consultation, including a second opinion, should be sought where the treating doctor has doubt about the proposed decision. In emergency medicine, procedures may be instituted which, when more information is available, appear unjustified. Where there is genuine doubt about the ability of a particular treatment to benefit the patient, that treatment should be provided but may be withdrawn if, on subsequent review, it is found to be inappropriate or not beneficial.

6. Withholding or withdrawing treatment

6.1 Although emotionally it may be easier to withhold treatment than to withdraw that which has been started, there are no legal, or necessary morally relevant, differences between the two actions.

The primary aim of instituting medical treatment is to provide a health benefit to the patient. The same justification is required for continuing treatment which has already been started. In fact, withdrawal of life-prolonging treatment is often morally safer than withholding it. In many cases the beneficial effects of such treatment cannot be foreseen, making it inappropriate to withhold treatment. Treatment is, therefore, often initiated in order to ascertain whether it is able to benefit the patient, even though it may subsequently be withdrawn when more information is available.

This view of the legal and moral equivalence of withholding and withdrawing treatment was expressed by Lord Goff and Lord Lowry in the *Bland* case, with the latter saying:

> *"I do not believe that there is a valid distinction between the omission to treat a patient and the abandonment of treatment which has been commenced, since to recognise such a distinction*

could quite illogically confer on a doctor who had refrained from treatment an immunity which did not benefit a doctor who had embarked on treatment in order to see whether it might help the patient and had abandoned the treatment when it was seen not to do so". [12]

In the Human Rights Act, public authorities are bound in relation to their omissions as well as their actions. [13]

Although there may be no legal or moral difference between withholding and withdrawing treatment when making decisions about an individual patient, this is not to say that emotionally and psychologically the two are equivalent. Many health professionals, as well as patients, feel an emotional difference between withholding and withdrawing treatment. This is likely to be linked to the largely negative impression attached to a decision to withdraw treatment which can be interpreted as abandonment or "giving up on the patient". The BMA considers that where a particular treatment is no longer benefiting the patient, continuing to provide it would not be in the patient's best interests and, indeed, might be thought to be morally wrong. Greater emphasis on the reasons for providing treatment (including artificial nutrition and hydration), rather than the justification for withholding it, and greater clarity about the legitimate scope and process of decision making by health professionals are likely to challenge this perceived difference.

6.2 Treatment should never be withheld, when there is a possibility that it will benefit the patient, simply because withholding is considered to be easier than withdrawing treatment.

There is a risk that the perceived difficulty of withdrawing treatment could lead to some patients failing to receive treatment which could benefit them. Where there is uncertainty about the benefit of a particular treatment, some health professionals may be reluctant to start treatment in the mistaken belief that, once initiated, the treatment cannot be withdrawn.

7.   How to use this guidance

7.1   This document is not an attempt to define rules which must be followed. Rather, it provides general guidance about the principles and factors to take into account in reaching a decision.

The term "guidance", rather than "protocol", has been chosen deliberately in this document to emphasise that it is an aid to the process of decision making rather than rules to be followed. This form of guidance does not provide a simple set of instructions to be followed without reflection but a tool to aid decision making; it does not provide easy answers but more an approach through which an appropriate decision may be reached. Although ultimately the responsibility and accountability rest with the doctor in charge of the patient's care, such decisions are increasingly made in a multidisciplinary setting. This document also provides a basis for discussion between health professionals and with the patient and those close to the patient.

PART 2   Decisions involving adults who have the capacity to make and communicate decisions or those who have a valid advance directive

8.   Medical assessment

8.1   All health care decisions, including decisions to withhold or withdraw life-prolonging treatment, should be based on the best available evidence. Relevant guidelines should be considered and additional specialist advice sought where appropriate.

Decisions taken by or with competent adult patients to withhold or withdraw life-prolonging treatment must be based on the best available medical evidence. This is also evident in the general duty to protect life to be found in Article 2 of the European Convention on Human Rights. Where relevant guidelines exist for the diagnosis and management of the condition, these should be consulted. Where there is reasonable doubt about the diagnosis or treatment options or where the health care team has limited experience of the condition, a further independent opinion should be sought. These issues are discussed in more detail in section 17.

9.   Contemporaneous refusals of life-prolonging treatment

9.1   A voluntary refusal of life-prolonging treatment by a competent adult must be respected.

It is well established in law and ethics that competent adults have the right to refuse any medical treatment, even if that refusal

15

results in their death. This position is reinforced by the Human Rights Act which is rooted in respect for the dignity of the person. Thus the Article 2 duty to protect life has to be balanced with the right to security of the person in Article 5 and the right to respect for privacy in Article 8. The patient is not obliged to justify his or her decision but the health team will usually wish to discuss the refusal with the patient in order to ensure that he or she has based that decision on accurate information and to correct any misunderstandings. Where the health team considers that the treatment would provide a net benefit, that assessment should be sympathetically explained to the patient but patients should not be pressured to accept treatment.

A refusal of a particular life-prolonging treatment does not imply a refusal of all treatment or all facets of basic care. The health team must continue to offer other treatments and all procedures which are solely or primarily intended to keep the patient comfortable and free from severe pain or discomfort. Procedures such as artificial nutrition and hydration and sedation may be refused by a patient who is competent to make that decision but they should continue to be available if the patient changes his or her mind. Their continued availability should be made clear to the patient at the time the original decision is made.

9.2   There is a legal presumption that adults have the competence to make decisions unless the contrary is proven.

The fact that an individual has made a decision which appears to others to be irrational or unjustified should not be taken as evidence that the individual lacks the mental capacity to make that decision. If, however, the decision is clearly contrary to previously expressed wishes or it is based on a misperception of reality such as, for example, believing that the blood is poisoned because it is red,[14] this may be indicative of a lack of the requisite capacity and further investigation will be required (see section 13.2).

9.3   Patients refusing medical treatment should have been offered information about the treatment proposed, the consequences of not having the treatment and any alternative forms of treatment available.

16

Patients refusing medical treatment should ideally base their decisions on sufficient accurate information including an awareness of the condition, the proposed treatment, any significant risks or side effects, the probability of a successful recovery, the consequences of not having the treatment and any alternative forms of treatment. Such information should always be offered but, legally, patients are not required to have accepted the offer of information in order for their refusal to be valid. It is important that the patient is given the opportunity to discuss the information if he or she wishes to do so.

9.4   Legally, to provide treatment for a competent adult without his or her consent, or in the face of a valid refusal, would constitute battery or assault and could result in legal action being taken against the doctor. It may also involve a breach of the patient's human rights. The law on battery and assault has traditionally applied even where the patient is a pregnant woman and her refusal would put the life of the fetus at risk as well as her own. However the right to life in Article 2 of the European Convention could, it has been suggested, extend to the unborn in certain circumstances so as to give the fetus, in some situations, a countervailing right to life. The law here is at present uncertain.

A competent adult's right to refuse treatment was reaffirmed in the 1998 case of *St George's Healthcare National Health Service Trust v S*[15] in which the court held that competent adults have the *absolute* right to refuse medical treatment (in that case a Caesarean section) even if they may die as a result of that refusal.

The European Court has avoided making a decision as to whether "everyone" includes the unborn child. Given that individual states are allowed a wide margin of appreciation on matters of a moral nature, discussion on the subject within the European Commission[16] and the way UK law has developed in this area, it is considered unlikely that a fetus would be considered, by the UK courts, to have legal rights under the Human Rights Act. Until a case has been considered, however, the law on this matter, particularly in relation to viable fetuses, will remain unclear.

10. Advance refusals of life-prolonging treatment

10.1 Where a patient has lost the capacity to make a decision but has a valid advance directive refusing life-prolonging treatment, this must be respected.

Increasingly patients are taking a more active role in their own health care and have clear views about what treatment they would or would not wish to be given. Many people fear that once they become incapable of making decisions, life-prolonging treatment may continue to be provided long after it is able to deliver a level of recovery, or length and quality of life, that they would find acceptable. Some people choose to express their views in the form of an advance statement which is made when the patient is competent but only becomes "active" once competence has been lost. Advance statements can cover a range of scenarios but one common subset of these, advance directives, refers specifically to advance refusals of treatment, including life-prolonging treatment. Advance directives are often presented as formalised written documents but it is not necessary for the refusal to be in writing in order to be valid. Frequently an individual will discuss his or her wishes with a general practitioner or another health professional and this may be recorded in the patient's notes. Where the discussion reflects a clear expression of the patient's wishes this will have the same status as a written advance directive, if that is the patient's intention.

Those considering making a formal advance directive should be aware of their disadvantages, as well as the benefits.[17] Where people choose to make an advance directive and the criteria for validity are met (see section 10.2), their views should be respected. Some advance directives name an individual the patient would wish the health care team to consult in making treatment decisions. Whilst the views of this person have no legal status and are not binding on the health care team (unless he or she has been formally appointed as proxy decision maker as is possible in Scotland, see section 13.4), previous discussions between the patient and this person may provide information which is useful in interpreting the directive. This can be particularly helpful where there is uncertainty or disagreement about the applicability of the directive to the circumstances which have arisen or where new treatments have been developed since the directive was drawn up.

Artificial nutrition and hydration may be one of the treatments rejected in an advance directive. Where the circumstances which have arisen are those envisaged by the patient, artificial nutrition and hydration should not be provided contrary to a clear advance refusal. The BMA does not, however, believe that advance refusals of basic care (see section 3.3), including the offer of oral nutrition and hydration and the offer of pain relief, should be binding on health professionals.

10.2 **In order for an advance refusal of treatment to be valid the patient must have been competent when the directive was made, must be acting free from pressure and must have been offered sufficient, accurate information to make an informed decision. The patient must also have envisaged the type of situation which has subsequently arisen and for which the advance directive is being invoked.**

The level of capacity required to refuse treatment in advance is the same level which would be required for making the decision contemporaneously. It is irrelevant whether the refusal is contrary to the views of most other people or whether the patient lacks insight into other aspects of his or her life. The courts upheld, for example, the rights of a Broadmoor patient with a psychotic disorder to refuse amputation of his gangrenous foot even though he held demonstrably erroneous views on other matters.[18] Judgments taking this line are likely to be reinforced by the Human Rights Act's emphasis on respect for the person and on his or her power of autonomous decision making.

In order to be valid, the directive must have envisaged the situation which has now arisen. Health professionals must use professional judgment to assess whether the refusal is applicable in the circumstances. In doing so, they should consult any individual nominated by the patient on the advance directive. If the refusal is not applicable to the circumstances, it will not be legally binding although it may still give valuable information about the individual's former wishes and values which can assist with decision making.

When health care teams are confronted with an incompetent adult who has an advance directive, and where time permits, further enquiries should be made to establish the validity of the document and to help to clarify the patient's intentions, for example, by speaking to those close to the patient and contacting the patient's general practitioner. Treatment should not be delayed, however, in order to look for an advance directive if there is no clear indication that one exists. Where there are good grounds for genuine doubt about the validity of an advance refusal, there should be a presumption in favour of life and emergency treatment should be provided. Treatment may, however, be withdrawn at a later stage should the validity, or existence, of a valid advance directive become clear.

10.3 A valid advance refusal of treatment has the same legal authority as a contemporaneous refusal and legal action could be taken against a doctor who provides treatment in the face of a valid refusal.

Although there is currently no statute on advance directives,[19] a number of legal cases have clearly established their legal status.[20] Any health professional who knowingly provides treatment in the face of a valid advance refusal may be liable to legal action for battery or assault and (following implementation of the Human Rights Act) a breach of the patient's human rights. Those close to the patient may be under the mistaken impression that they have the power to override an advance directive and health professionals complying with a valid advance directive should explain to the relatives their reasons for doing so.

10.4 More detailed information about advance refusals can be found in the BMA's code of practice, *Advance Statements About Medical Treatment*.[21]

11. Contemporaneous requests for life-prolonging treatment

11.1 Although patients' wishes should always be discussed with them, the fact that a patient has requested a particular treatment does not mean that it must always be provided. The positive duty on health

professionals to protect life, which is to be found in Article 2 of the European Convention, does not go this far.

(a)   Health professionals are not obliged to provide any treatment which cannot produce the desired benefit.

Treatment is usually considered unable to produce the desired benefit either because it cannot achieve its physiological aim or because the burdens of the treatment are considered to outweigh the benefits for the particular individual. (This is sometimes called "futile" treatment.) Where the individual is competent, he or she should be offered a full discussion about the likely outcome of the treatment; if the patient refuses this offer, his or her wish not to have information should be respected. The patient's own view about the acceptable level of burden or risk, where this is known, will carry considerable weight in assessing the overall benefit of the treatment to the patient. It is questionable whether a treatment could be considered to be of no "benefit" to the patient – given a broad definition of benefit – if the patient knows, and has accepted, the chance and level of expected recovery and wishes to accept treatment on that basis.

Sometimes patients may request all treatment, despite the profound risks or side effects which would seem to most people to outweigh the small, or short-lived, potential benefit. This may be because of a willingness to accept any level of risk in the hope of prolonging life, an unstinting belief in the ability of medicine to cure all ills or an inability to come to terms with the full implications of their condition. Whilst it may not be acceptable to continue to provide treatment indefinitely, which is unable to produce the desired benefit, there are strong arguments for complying with reasonable requests from competent patients for treatment to be continued for a limited period to allow them to achieve a particular goal or to sort out their affairs. What is "reasonable" will need to be judged on an individual basis, taking account of factors such as the patient's ability to achieve the goal, the time it would take to do so and the potential opportunity costs for other patients who may be denied treatment as a consequence of respecting the patient's wishes. Taking account of these and other relevant factors, the decision of whether to provide treatment will ultimately be made by the clinician in charge of the patient's care with advice from the rest of the health care team. The courts have made clear on many occasions that doctors are not obliged to provide treatment contrary to their clinical judgment[22] and it is extremely unlikely that the duty to protect life in Article 2 of the European Convention will be construed in a way which undermines this clear principle. Where treatment is withheld or withdrawn, this will require careful discussion with the patient who is likely to require ongoing support to help him or her come to terms with the situation. Such discussion, or at least the creation of an opportunity for such discussion, should also be regarded as part of a patient's right to respect for his or her private life under Article 8 of the European Convention.

> **(b)   There is no obligation to provide any treatment which is clearly contrary to an individual's health interests. A life-prolonging treatment may, for example, prolong life but result in severe pain or loss of function so that overall it produces extreme harm to the patient.**

Sometimes patients request treatment or medical procedures which are contrary to their own health interests. Such a situation might arise with an experimental procedure which has a very low chance of success but a very high chance of harm. Whilst patients may be willing to take any chance in order to prolong life, the health care team is not obliged to comply with such requests. In such situations, the team should also be mindful of the duty under Article 3 of the European Convention not to subject anyone to inhuman or degrading treatment.

> **(c)   Except in an emergency situation, doctors are not obliged to treat contrary to their conscience (although they may be obliged to make an appropriate referral).**

Where a health professional has a conscientious objection to a particular procedure or action, such as the termination of pregnancy, even though it might be life-prolonging for the patient, he or she should transfer care of the patient to a colleague. If, however, the procedure is required immediately in order to save the patient's life and no suitable colleague is available, the doctor must provide appropriate treatment. This position is reinforced by the right to freedom of conscience and religion which is to be found in Article 9 of the European Convention, which is however subject to restriction where "necessary in a democratic society" for, among other reasons, "the protection of health" and the "protection of ... the rights and freedoms of others".

(d) Where resources are limited, it is inevitable that some patients will not receive all of the treatment they request even though such treatment could potentially benefit them.

Increasing levels of technology have not only presented ethical dilemmas about assessing when treatment ceases to benefit the patient but have also raised the issue of withholding or withdrawing potentially beneficial treatment on grounds of cost. Where funds are limited, individual hospitals, doctors and patients are competing for resources. Particular difficulties could arise if, for example, a patient requests life-prolonging treatment to be continued for as long as technically possible, even though there is no hope of recovery. Complying with such a request could be at the expense of another patient who has a reasonable chance of recovery if treatment is provided. For example, a doctor is not obliged to comply with a request for intensive care and all treatment and procedures which could potentially prolong the life of a patient who is dying from cancer. The doctor may, however, be willing to provide treatment for a limited period to enable the patient to achieve some particular goal or to sort out his or her affairs. Health professionals have an ethical duty to make the best use of the available resources and this means that hard decisions must be made. Whilst this is a much broader issue than can be discussed thoroughly in this document, it is clear that doctors are not obliged to comply with patients' requests for treatment when they make inequitable demands on scarce resources. It is improbable that the courts will turn Article 2's guarantee of the right to life into a positive obligation to supply treatment regardless of cost.[23] However, special care should be taken to avoid making such decisions on a discriminatory basis which cannot subsequently be objectively justified. Such a practice could involve a breach of the European Convention's prohibition (in Article 14) of discrimination in the enjoyment of the rights that appear in the Convention.

12. Advance requests for life-prolonging treatment

12.1 There is no obligation to comply with advance requests for life-prolonging treatment but these should be taken into account in assessing the patient's best interests. The same exceptions would apply as for contemporaneous decisions (see section 11).

As well as the actual wording of an advance request for life-prolonging treatment, the general spirit and tone of the statement should also be taken into account. The same exceptions apply as to contemporaneous requests although the lack of opportunity for discussion with the patient, for example about what level of recovery would justify the burdens of the treatment for that person, makes decision making in these circumstances more difficult.

PART 3 Decisions involving adults who do not have the capacity to make or communicate decisions and do not have a valid advance directive and decisions involving children and young people

PART 3A Decisions involving adults

13. Capacity and incapacity

13.1 There is a legal presumption that adults have the competence to make decisions unless the contrary is proven. Where there are grounds for doubting competence (see section 9.2), further investigation will be required.

13.2 People have varying levels of capacity and should be encouraged to participate in discussion and decision making about all aspects of their lives to the greatest extent possible. The graver the consequences of the decision, the commensurately greater the level of competence required to take that decision.

Capacity is often discussed as though it is something which patients either definitively have or lack but the boundary is often less certain.[24] People have varying levels of capacity and an individual's capacity may fluctuate over time. An individual may have the capacity to express preferences, such as about where to live, for example, but not to refuse life-prolonging treatment. At the other end of the scale, some individuals may be totally unable to make any decisions either because of profound intellectual impairment, the loss of any ability to communicate or unconsciousness. The level of capacity required to make a decision will depend upon the consequences of the decision being taken. A greater level of understanding and competence will be required to refuse life-prolonging treatment than will be necessary, for example, to refuse a flu vaccination. Patients who have not attained the required level should still, where possible, be involved in discussion about treatment options even though their views may not be determinative. Where there is genuine uncertainty about an individual's capacity to refuse life-prolonging treatment, advice should be sought from a psychiatrist or an appropriately experienced chartered clinical psychologist. The role of these professionals is to assess the patient's capacity to give valid consent. They cannot give consent on behalf of the patient and only treatment for a mental disorder may be authorised under mental health legislation.[25]

The case of *Re MB*[26] provided clarification from the courts that an individual may lack capacity where:

- he or she is unable to comprehend and retain the information which is material to the decision, especially as to the likely consequences of having the treatment in question;
- he or she is unable to use the information and weigh it in the balance as part of the process of arriving at a decision.

Individuals should be given practical assistance to maximise their decision making capacity. This should include providing information in broad terms and simple language, including material translated into other languages if appropriate, and other modes of communication such as video or audio cassette. Patients should not be regarded as incapable of making or communicating a decision unless all practical steps have been taken to maximise their ability to do so.[27] For some patients, however, such as those with advanced dementia, in a coma or persistent vegetative state, all decision making capacity is clearly lacking.

13.3 At present in England, Wales and Northern Ireland no other individual has the power to give or withhold consent for the treatment of an adult who lacks decision making capacity but treatment may be provided, without consent, if it is considered by the clinician in charge of the patient's care to be necessary and in the best interests of the patient.

There is a widely held misperception that the next of kin may give, or withhold, consent on behalf of an adult patient who lacks the capacity to make or communicate decisions. In fact, no such legal power is given to the next of kin or to those with enduring power of attorney although the Government has proposed the introduction of a new system of decision making for mentally incapacitated adults (information regarding any changes to the law will be put on the BMA's website). Currently, decisions about whether to provide, withhold or withdraw treatment are the responsibility of the treating doctor with the advice of the rest of the health care team and with reference to the courts in particularly contentious, difficult or disputed cases. Clearly however, being mindful of the duty of confidentiality, it is right to consult with appropriate family members under such circumstances, and this may also be required under the Human Rights Act, with its obligation on public authorities to respect a person's private and family life under Article 8 of the European Convention. In the case of *Re F* [28] the courts clarified that treatment may be provided to an incompetent adult where that treatment is necessary ("action properly taken to preserve the life, health or well-being of the assisted person") and in the patient's best interests. By its very nature, the provision of life-prolonging treatment will preserve the life of the patient but it may not be in the patient's best interests. Where the treatment is not benefiting the patient, in a broad sense, the justification for providing the treatment does not exist and treatment cannot lawfully be provided. Therefore, decisions to provide treatment, including artificial nutrition and hydration, need to be justified.

13.4 In Scotland a proxy decision maker may be appointed to give consent to medical treatment on behalf of an incapacitated person over 16 years of age.

The Adults with Incapacity (Scotland) Act allows the appointment of a proxy decision maker (a guardian, welfare attorney or person authorised under an intervention order) who is entitled to give consent to the medical treatment of an incapacitated patient over the age of 16.[29] Where such a proxy is appointed, he or she must be consulted (where reasonable and practicable) about proposed medical treatment. The Act also puts on a statutory footing the authority of doctors to do what is reasonable in the circumstances to safeguard or promote an incapacitated patient's physical or mental health where no proxy has been appointed.

If there is disagreement between the doctor in charge of the patient's care and the proxy decision maker, the doctor must ask the Mental Welfare Commission to nominate a doctor to provide a second opinion. Where that nominated doctor agrees that treatment should be given, the treating doctor may provide treatment notwithstanding the disagreement of the proxy. Whatever the nominated doctor's opinion about the treatment, the treating doctor, proxy or any other person with an interest in the personal welfare of the patient may apply to the court of Session for a determination as to whether the proposed treatment should be given or not. The Act leaves open the option for ministers to define specific treatments which should be handled outwith this regime. At the time of writing, no treatments had been so specified.

The Act covers decisions about the provision of treatment and not decisions to withdraw or withhold treatment. The court's inherent jurisdiction to give consent to or refuse medical treatment for incapacitated adults and children has been held to entitle it to authorise the withdrawal of treatment from a patient for whom continued treatment does not provide a benefit.

In addition to its clear proxy decision making powers, the Act also requires doctors to take account of the views of the nearest relative and primary carer of the adult and doctors are advised to do so, bearing in mind the duty of confidentiality to the patient. This may also be required under the Human Rights Act.

13.5 Where patients have lost the capacity to make decisions, their past wishes, values and preferences should be taken into account in making treatment decisions.

Part of the assessment of whether a particular treatment would provide a benefit to the patient is to consider whether the extent of recovery which might be achieved would be considered acceptable to the individual patient, if he or she were able to express a view. Where the individual is incompetent and has not made a clear advance declaration of wishes, this involves taking account of any previously expressed views or preferences or the values which were important to the individual when competent. This is unlikely to provide sufficient information to give a definitive answer but it can be helpful as part of the broader decision making process. It is also within the spirit of Article 9 of the European Convention which emphasises the importance of freedom of thought, conscience and religion.

13.6 Where the patient has never attained even a minimal level of capacity, decision making is more difficult. In these cases the primary factor will be the clinical benefits and burdens of treatment.

Where the patient has never had capacity and has therefore been unable to express any views about the circumstances under which life-prolonging treatment might be refused, or to provide any indication of those aspects of life which are valued, health professionals must rely on other factors in making decisions. Whilst acknowledging that decisions in such circumstances are likely to be influenced by subjective responses, it is important for the health care team to be constantly aware that the primary consideration is whether the perceived benefits of the treatment would outweigh the burdens to the patient, not whether the health care team, or the patient's relatives or carers, would wish to have treatment themselves in that situation. Although the decision rests with the clinician in charge of the patient's care, the views of those responsible for the continuing care of the patient, which would include those close to the patient, should form an important part of that assessment. Care should always be taken to ensure that such decisions are made on an individual basis and that no unjustifiable discrimination occurs.

13.7 The same principles apply when decisions are taken in relation to a woman who is pregnant with a viable

fetus and is unable to make or communicate decisions. Traditionally under UK law the fetus has no legal status and the decision must be that which represents the best interests of the pregnant woman. The extent to which the woman's likely wishes about the outcome of the pregnancy may be taken into account in determining her best interests is unclear. In order that these matters may be fully explored, legal advice should be sought. In particular it remains to be clarified whether the fetus has Convention rights (in particular the right to life (Article 2) and the right not to be discriminated against (Article 14)) which would be required to be balanced against those of the mother (see section 9.4).

PART 3B   Decisions involving babies, children and young people

14.   Duties owed to babies, children and young people

14.1   **The same moral duties are owed to babies, children and young people as to adults and the considerations, process and safeguards proposed in Parts 3C and 3D of this document apply to both adults and children.**

14.2   **As with adults, the patient's best interests and an assessment of the benefits and burdens of treatment are the key factors in considering whether treatment should be provided or withdrawn.**

The BMA believes that the high standards set for decision making with and for adults apply similarly to decisions in paediatric care. Although specific and important differences exist between adult and child patients, the ethical principles which underlie the provision or continuation of treatment, namely that it should only proceed where it would provide a net benefit to the patient, hold for all.

From birth, all people have the right to expect appropriate care and decisions must be taken in a way which is perceived to reflect their best interests or, where this is not achievable, which is not contrary to their interests. Misperceptions may have arisen, however, as a result of societal acceptance of termination of pregnancy in cases of serious handicap. Some people, including some parents of babies born with congenital abnormalities, believe that a willingness for late termination of pregnancy because of serious handicap means that more leeway should be allowed regarding withholding or withdrawing life-prolonging treatment from handicapped newborns than from similarly impaired older babies, children or adults. Enquiries to the BMA appear to indicate that some doctors consider that if parental agreement is obtained, they need not provide life-sustaining treatment for babies born with a severe impairment. This perceived difference also applies to older children with evidence from America suggesting that:

> *"clinicians frequently give young patients more chances to revive from and survive their illnesses than they offer to older, particularly elderly patients. Clinicians also seem more willing to impose greater burdens on children with fewer chances of success than on adults".*[30]

Legally and ethically, decisions to treat or not to treat are justifiable only where this is in the child's best interests. But reasons for differences in perception may be significant and require further analysis. Willingness to continue with treatment may reflect the fact that a decision to stop striving to maintain life is emotionally more difficult to make for children than adults or that outcomes may be less predictable for children due to a small evidence base from which to judge the likely outcome. The developmental potential of children is also important and paediatricians will consider the quality of this potential for progression from incompetence to competence as a factor in decision making.

The BMA believes that the ethical underpinnings of paediatric, adult and geriatric medicine are the same and articulates the principles it considers relevant to any decisions about cessation of treatment in this document. The additional and particular issues which arise for babies, children and young people are addressed in this section.[31]

These guidelines emphasise that where there is reasonable uncertainty about the benefit of life-prolonging treatment, there should be a presumption in favour of initiating it, although there are circumstances in which active intervention (other than basic care) would not be appropriate since best interests is not synonymous with prolongation of life. Criteria for deciding best interests are the same as those for adults; including whether the child has the potential to develop awareness, the ability to interact and the capacity for self-directed action and whether the child will suffer severe unavoidable pain and distress.

If the child's condition is incompatible with survival or where there is broad consensus that the condition is so severe that treatment would not provide a benefit in terms of being able to restore or maintain the patient's health, intervention may be unjustified. Similarly, where treatments would involve suffering or distress to the child, these and other burdens must be weighed against the anticipated benefit, even if life cannot be prolonged without treatment.

This view was confirmed by the courts in the 1990 case of *Re J*.[32] Baby J was born very prematurely and was severely brain damaged. He appeared to be blind and was expected to be deaf and unlikely ever to be able to speak or develop even limited intellectual abilities. Despite these disabilities he was thought to feel pain in the same way as other babies. His life expectancy was uncertain and he required repeated, invasive procedures to keep him alive. The court held that to continue such invasive treatments would not be in his best interests and treatment need not be given when the patient "suffered from physical disabilities so grave that his life would from *his point of view* be so intolerable" that if he were able to make a sound judgment, he would not choose treatment.

Where there is clinical uncertainty about whether specific treatments should be considered, because it is unclear whether they provide sufficient benefit to outweigh the burdens, the BMA believes that it is particularly important that parents are frankly informed of that. Parents are generally the best judges of their young children's, and the family's, interests but they need full, clear and accurate information including about the general likelihood of success and also the doctor's own success rates for the particular type of treatment or procedure. Doctors, children and informed parents share the decision, with doctors taking the lead in judging the clinical factors and parents the lead on determining best interests more generally. The views of the various parties can, however, be challenged. If disagreement is unresolved, ultimately a court may provide guidance or assistance in determining whether the provision of life-prolonging treatment would benefit the child. The court is required to pay particular regard to the welfare of the child,[33] and guidance on what factors should be considered is given in the 1989 Children Act:

"(a) *the ascertainable wishes and feelings of the child concerned (considered in the light of his age and understanding);*

(b) *his physical, emotional and educational needs;*

(c) *the likely effect on him of any change in his circumstances;*

(d) *his age, sex, background and any characteristics of his which the court considers relevant;*

(e) *any harm which he has suffered or is at risk of suffering; [and]*

(f) *how capable each of his parents, and any other person in relation to whom the court considers the question to be relevant, is of meeting his needs".*

Courts will also need to consider the child's human rights including whether the proposed treatment involves the possibility of subjecting the child to inhuman or degrading treatment, in contravention of Article 3 of the European Convention.

Children's roles in determining what their interests are and whether treatment would provide a benefit for them increase as their maturity and ability to express views develop. They should always be encouraged and helped to understand the treatment and care they are receiving and to participate in decision making to the extent they are willing and able to do so.

Where a decision is reached to withhold or withdraw a particular treatment, it is essential to emphasise that this does not represent abandonment or "giving up" on the child but a realisation that continued treatment would not be in the child's best interests. It is the value of the *treatment* which is being assessed, not the value of the *child*. Although the immediate goal may, rightly, have shifted from seeking the benefits which arise from prolonging life to seeking those which arise from being comfortable and free from pain, the overall objective of providing benefit does not change.

15. Decision making for babies and young children who cannot consent for themselves

15.1 Those with parental responsibility for a baby or young child are legally and morally entitled to give or withhold consent to treatment. Their decisions will usually be determinative unless they conflict seriously with the interpretation of those providing care about the child's best interests.

The fundamental legal difference between decisions for adults and children is the ability of another person to authorise a particular course of treatment or non-treatment, provided that this is in the child's best interests. Although the BMA believes it is always important to involve those close to the patient in decision making, both legally and morally the influence of their views will be stronger where the patient is a baby or young child.

People with parental responsibility[34] for babies and young children have the legal power to give or withhold consent to treatment for a child, provided that they are not acting against his or her best interests and are acting on the basis of accurate information. This is the way the law balances the right to life of the child with the respect for family privacy and freedom of conscience which are to be found in Article 8 and Article 9 of the European Convention respectively. Where there is genuine uncertainty about which treatment option would be of most clinical benefit, parents are usually best placed and equipped to weigh this evidence and apply it to their child's own circumstances. They need to do this in conjunction with medical advice and the decisions of parents and doctors together should determine what course of action is to be followed. All reasonable options should be discussed with the parents, although the actual treatment decision will depend on the medical assessment of benefit.

As with all other patients, where there is uncertainty about whether the treatment is in a child's best interests, it may be appropriate to initiate treatment for a trial period with a subsequent review. This allows for the effectiveness of the treatment to be assessed and can help to stabilise the child's condition to allow time for further appraisal of the situation. This is vitally important when there has not been sufficient opportunity to discuss treatment options with the parents, for example in the labour ward. Where the parents hold strong views in favour of either withdrawing or continuing treatment, these, together with the reasons for their views, should be given serious consideration as part of the decision making process. Taking these decisions can be distressing and burdensome for parents and the health care team should offer support. Some parents may ask the doctor to make the decision.

Children with insufficient maturity and understanding to make treatment decisions for themselves are often able to express views or opinions about their care. Ideally children should be encouraged to talk about what is happening to them, so that they are given the opportunity to understand their illness and treatment. Their preferences on issues such as when to receive treatment, and where, should be taken into account and should influence decisions whenever possible. Children can also be encouraged to feel involved by allowing them to take other, easier, decisions, such as who should accompany them during treatment.

Parents' powers to withhold consent for a child's treatment is likely to be curtailed where the treatment refused would provide a clear benefit to the child, where the statistical chances of recovery are good or where the severity and burdens of the condition are not sufficient to justify withholding or withdrawing life-prolonging treatment. If parents and doctors do not agree after sufficient discussion and time has been taken, a second opinion should be sought. In some cases, where agreement cannot be reached, the matter may have to go to court (see section 15.3).

15.2 The law has confirmed that best interests and the balance of benefits and burdens are essential components of decision making and that the views of parents are a part of this. However, parents cannot necessarily insist on enforcing decisions based solely on their own preferences where these conflict with good medical evidence.

While the decision of parents will usually be the factor determining treatment, parents cannot legally or ethically insist upon treatment which the health care team considers to be inappropriate or when the burdens of the treatment clearly outweigh the benefits for the child. Whilst it is entirely understandable for parents to want to prolong their child's life for as long as possible, the BMA's view, as stated elsewhere, is that:

> *"for desperate parents to expose fatally ill children to all manner of painful, unproven or essentially futile treatments breaches the child's right to be free from intrusion. The doctor's first duty is to the patient and in such cases the main task may involve helping the family face reality. Family pressure to provide aggressive intervention of dubious clinical value should be resisted"*.[35]

Wherever possible, decisions should be taken at a pace comfortable to those involved, allowing time for discussion, explanation and reflection so that decisions are informed and reflective of the child's best interests and so those close to the child have time to consult others close to them and adjust to their decisions. It may be useful to bring in additional clinical expertise and to seek further medical opinions and parents may benefit from the opportunity to speak to other parents who have been through similar experiences. Sooner or later, however, a time will come when a decision has to be made about whether treatment should be continued and, if the parents and health care team are still unable to agree, it would be advisable to seek legal advice.

15.3 If agreement cannot be reached some form of legal review may be required.

Parents and the health care team will usually reach agreement over what is best for a child patient. Their goal is the same – to benefit the child – and in the vast majority of cases their views about how this can be achieved will coincide.

However, if agreement cannot be reached in a reasonable time period, which will depend on the nature and likely course of the child's condition, it may be necessary to seek legal review and ask the courts for guidance on what is best for a particular child. As the legal system in the UK is an adversarial one, seeking judicial opinion may be upsetting for all concerned and it is essential that ongoing support is provided for the parents, other relatives and those involved with treating and caring for the child. The BMA believes that less confrontational means of problem solving are preferable.

If the child has been made a ward of court, a decision must not be made about withholding or withdrawing treatment without seeking authorisation from the court.

In exceptional cases, the courts have been willing to authorise the withholding or withdrawing of life-prolonging treatment, against the parents' wishes, where it was considered that continued treatment would be contrary to the child's best interests. In 1997, for example, the High Court endorsed a doctor's decision to withhold artificial ventilation and refrain from resuscitating a 16-month-old girl with a desperately serious disease.[36] Baby C was suffering from spinal muscular atrophy type 1, a disease which causes severe emaciation and disability. The judge described the parents as highly responsible, religious orthodox Jews, who loved their daughter but who were unable to "bring themselves to face the inevitable future". The doctor's treatment plan of withholding resuscitation and ventilation and providing palliative care was endorsed by the judge to "ease the suffering of this little girl to allow her life to end peacefully".

Shortly before the implementation of the Human Rights Act, the courts heard a similar case, in which a health care team sought approval to withhold artificial ventilation from a baby boy despite the objection of his parents.[37] Referring back to previous cases in which non-treatment had been found to be in the best interests of the child, the High Court held that it would be lawful for artificial ventilation to be withheld if, in the opinion of the treating paediatrician, that was clinically appropriate. The judge went on to say that withholding this treatment did not conflict with any Article of the European Convention. The judge was of the view that there could be no infringement of the right to life (Article 2) because withholding artificial ventilation was in the baby's best interests, and the right to be free from inhuman or degrading treatment (Article 3) included a right to dignity in death.

The courts have also upheld a parent's refusal against the advice of doctors. In 1996, the case of *Re T*[38] was heard by the courts. T suffered from biliary atresia and was not expected to live beyond two and a half years without a liver transplant. He had had major invasive and unsuccessful surgery at three and a half weeks old, which had appeared to cause him severe pain and distress. His mother did not want to expose her son to further distress and believed that it would be best for him to be cared for by her abroad, where T's father was working.

Lord Justice Waite made the point, which the BMA endorses, that:

> *"the greater the scope for genuine debate between one view and another [about the best interests of the child], the stronger will be the inclination of the court to be influenced by a reflection that in the last analysis the best interests of every child include an expectation that difficult decisions affecting the length and quality of its life will be taken for it by the parent to whom its care has been entrusted by nature".*

This decision makes clear the importance and impact of a broad understanding of best interests. The case illustrates the validity and weight the courts have given to parents' assessment of their children's best interests and how the broad effects on the family can be a factor in these interests. Where decisions are finely balanced and it is not clear what would be best for a child, the view of parents should be determinative although difficulties may arise if the parents themselves disagree. A consequence of reliance on these factors is the possibility that two patients with the same clinical presentation could be treated differently provided that it could be shown that the parents were fulfilling their duty of care.

It must be noted that the cases that reach court are not typical and inevitably reflect the extreme situations in which prior agreement has not been reached.

16. Decision making by competent minors

16.1 A young person who has sufficient competence and understanding of the proposed treatment may give a valid consent regardless of age. A refusal of treatment by a young person under the age of 18, however, may not be determinative.

Any young person under the age of 18, who has a sufficient level of competence and understanding, can independently seek medical advice and give valid consent to treatment. The law[39] requires that he or she has sufficient understanding and intelligence to enable him or her to understand fully what is proposed and that provided young people do, their consent provides the necessary legal authorisation for treatment to go ahead. Young people should be encouraged to identify their own wants and needs and also to involve their parents and others close to them in decisions.

In English law, there is no automatic assumption of competence for people under 16[40] and those providing the treatment must make an assessment in each case. The assessment must look at the individual's understanding of the condition and the proposed treatment and of the consequences of any decision which is made. The test for competence is functional – whether somebody has capacity to do something depends on what that something is – and so for all patients the gravity of the decision plays an important part in the assessment of whether consent is valid. For example, the level of competence required to take a relatively straightforward decision about whether to have a broken arm set is not as great as that which is required to decide whether or not to have chemotherapy where the chances of its success are less than optimal. The importance of this has been seen in the courts' handling of refusals of life-prolonging treatment by teenagers (see section 16.2).

Young people can have high levels of maturity and understanding in relation to their illness and it is important not to prejudge them according to age. The BMA notes proposals to set an age far lower than 16 at which competence should be assumed. A presumption of competence set at compulsory school age has been proposed[41] and it has also been suggested[42] that at 9 years of age children begin to have the competence to agree to participate in research in a meaningful way. However, it is also often recommended that there is a duty to assess the competence of each individual child.[43] The BMA believes that rather than setting a particular age at which competence should be presumed, health professionals should be aware of the potential participatory abilities of all children and assess each individual child for the decisions in question. Children who have lived with disability or ongoing treatment for a particular condition, for example, or have experienced people close to them suffering in a similar way usually have a much higher level of understanding and insight than others who lack such personal experience.

16.2   Treatment in a young person's best interests may proceed where there is consent from somebody authorised to give it: the competent young person him or herself, somebody with parental responsibility or a court. It is unclear whether a young person's refusal can, in law, take precedence over the consent of either parents or a court.

Legal differences between England, Wales and Northern Ireland and Scotland demand that the issue of consent to treatment by minors be dealt with separately.

England, Wales and Northern Ireland

In legal terms, consent from a competent young person allows doctors to proceed to treat him or her. A person is presumed to be competent to make medical decisions at the age of 16[44] and it would be for others to establish that he or she was not competent. Below that age, as the judgment in *Gillick*[45] established, a young person may be deemed to be competent to make the decision in question. Where a competent young person consents to proposed treatment, it is not necessary to have parental consent in addition to that of the young person. Indeed, treatment may proceed against the wishes of the parents.[46]

Although competent young people can in law give a valid consent to treatment, it does not necessarily follow that they have the same right to refuse treatment. In legal cases heard before the implementation of the Human Rights Act, the courts made clear that parents and courts did not lose their right to give consent on behalf of a young person under the age of 18. It is possible that the Human Rights Act may change the outcome of such cases in the future.

As Lord Donaldson put it:

> *"[a Gillick competent] child can consent, but if he or she declines to do so or refuses, consent can be given by someone else who has parental rights or responsibilities. The failure or refusal of the Gillick competent child is a very important factor in the doctor's*

decision whether or not to treat, but does not prevent the necessary consent being obtained from another competent source".[47]

Case law involving young people's refusals of treatment has so far dealt with extreme or particularly complex situations, where the treatment being proposed is life-saving, and often there have been doubts about competence. In the case where Lord Donaldson's comments were made, the young person, R, was a 15-year-old ward of court who refused antipsychotic treatment. She had poor and sometimes violent relationships with her parents and appeared to experience visual and auditory hallucinations and sometimes suicidal thoughts. But she also experienced periods of lucidity, during which her doctors thought that she did have the competence to make decisions about her treatment. The court decided to authorise treatment to proceed, even against her wishes. In the circumstances, because the periods of R's competence were fluctuating, the court decided that she was not competent according to the standards set out in *Gillick*.

In another case of refusal, W[48] was 16 years old and under local authority care when her physical condition due to anorexia nervosa deteriorated to the extent that the authority wished to transfer her to hospital for treatment. W appeared capable of understanding the information given to her and what would be the consequence of not receiving treatment but refused to accept it. Her refusal was, however, overridden with the argument that it was symptomatic of her condition which involved a desire not to be treated. Therefore, again, the basis of the decision reached was that the young person was not in fact competent to refuse treatment. However, the court was strongly of the view that even if she had been deemed to be competent, treatment would have been authorised to proceed because it was in her best interests. It was here stated that a refusal of treatment by a young person up to the age of 18, even if that person was competent, could be overridden if consent was given by a parent or a court, provided that the treatment was in the young person's best interests. Whether this overriding of the wishes of a competent person under 18 will be seen to be compatible with such a person's Convention rights to security of the person (Article 5), respect for privacy (Article 8), freedom of conscience (Article 9) and non-discrimination in the enjoyment of these rights (Article 14) is an issue certain to come before the courts sooner or later. Any doctor who finds him or herself in such a situation should seek legal advice.

Even before the Human Rights Act, judgments in these cases and the development of the law in relation to refusals of life-prolonging treatment by competent young people, have been controversial. It is arguable that a right to consent is meaningless without a corresponding right to refuse and that the courts have adopted a strict test in determining necessary competence which even patients for whom competence is assumed (those over 16) are unlikely to satisfy.[49] The BMA believes that "minors who are clearly competent to agree to treatment must be acknowledged as also having an option to refuse treatment if they understand the implications of so doing".[50] It is accepted that the level of competence necessary to validly refuse life-prolonging treatment is very high but the BMA hopes that the exploration of treatment options and young people's wishes and values will allow agreement to be reached.

Since their refusals of treatment may not determine their care, the advance refusal of young people will not carry the same weight as the advance refusals of competent adults. However, as with any expression of wishes, advance refusals can play a part in the decision making process.

Scotland

In Scotland, the law has developed somewhat differently. As in England, Wales and Northern Ireland, the presumption of competence over 16 years of age is enshrined in statute but in Scotland the legislation also makes specific provision to allow people under 16 to validly consent provided they are "capable of understanding the nature and possible consequences of the procedure or treatment".[51] Additionally, the Children (Scotland) Act 1995 provides that a person may act as a child's legal representative (for example, by giving consent to medical treatment) only if the child is not capable of doing so on his or her own behalf. Thus the concurrent authority of competent young people, their parents and courts to consent, which is present in English law, is absent in Scottish law.

There has been little case law on the interpretation of this matter and at the time of writing, only one case had been reported. In that case, the Court of First Instance upheld the right of a competent 15-year-old boy to refuse medical treatment and confirmed that his mother's consent could not authorise the treatment. However, the medical treatment being proposed was for mental illness and the court ordered that he could, and in this case should, be formally detained under section 18 of the Mental Health (Scotland) Act 1984 to receive the treatment which was considered medically necessary. While this case was finally dealt with on the basis of the mental condition of the boy, it was necessary to use the statute only because the court decided that the boy's refusal of treatment for his mental illness was legally valid and could not be overridden by his mother. If the proposed treatment had not been for a condition covered by the mental health legislation, presumably treatment could not have been authorised. The argument whether the court itself could override his refusal of consent was not directly addressed but from the reasoning given by the court, it would seem that this would have been open to the same objections as invalidated the consent of the mother.

The cases which have been brought before the English courts on refusal of treatment have almost invariably involved young people who were deemed to lack the competence to take such grave decisions and often a degree of mental impairment was a feature of the case. Although the situation in Scotland appears to offer more autonomy to young people, it must be remembered that the young person must still be deemed to be competent to make the particular decision. Once the young person meets this criterion, it seems likely that his or her decision cannot be overridden by either parents or courts, whether the decision is to accept or reject treatment. However, this point may not be regarded as being settled.

16.3   Even where they are not determinative, the views and wishes of competent young people are an essential component of the assessment of their best interests and should, therefore, be given serious consideration at all stages of decision making.

Young people should be encouraged to be involved in decisions about their health care to a degree with which they are comfortable and the law requires that their views be heard.[52] Information cannot be forced upon unwilling recipients but older children benefit from having their wishes heard without having to accept the full responsibility of decision making alone. If a young person refuses treatment, time should be taken to explore the reasons for this and to ensure that any misunderstandings that might be present are corrected.

Doctors should also consider what impact complying with a young person's refusal would have on his or her longer term chances of survival, improvement or recovery. For example, young people who have had repeated chemotherapy which has not provided a significant improvement, and for whom there is uncertainty about the chance of achieving therapeutic benefit, may decide that they do not wish to repeat it. When deciding what is in young people's best interests, having weighed the likelihood of clinical success, such refusals may tip the balance in favour of withholding further treatments.

Doctors are reluctant to force competent young people to have treatment against their will, even on the hypothesis that the treatment would be lawful because appropriate consent has been given. Clearly the imperative to provide treatment weakens as the benefit it provides is less critical or its likelihood of success is smaller. Where non-treatment would be life-threatening or postponement would lead to serious and permanent injury, moral arguments for providing it against a young person's will are stronger than if the procedure proposed is elective or the consequences of not providing it are less grave.

In addition to being difficult to achieve in practice and possibly unlawful, forcing competent young people to undergo treatment where they refuse could be damaging to the young person's current and future relationship with health care givers and could undermine trust in the medical profession.[53] Whilst such considerations may not be determinative, the effects on competent young people of overriding their wishes must be considered in assessment of their best interests.

Young people should be given information as to any possibility there might be that their refusal may be overridden; for example if their parents consent, if a court authorises treatment or treatment is provided under mental health legislation.

PART 3C   The process of decision making for children and adults who lack the ability to make or communicate decisions

17.   Medical factors to be considered

17.1   For all patients treatment decisions, including those to withhold or withdraw life-prolonging treatment, must be based on the best available clinical evidence.

Factual information should be collected about the patient's condition, diagnosis and prognosis including the stability of the patient's condition over a period of time and the underlying pathology. Wherever possible, the assessment of the patient's condition should be evidence based and carried out according to best practice. However reliably evidence based, treatment decisions will inevitably be made on the balance of probabilities in the individual case. In assessing the medical information available, important factors are opinions about the accuracy of the diagnosis or prognosis and the degree of unavoidable uncertainty.

It is vital that research findings on treatment outcomes are made widely available and that, through continuing professional education, doctors ensure that they keep up to date with new developments. Doctors also have obligations to undergo a process of revalidation of their skills both for their own protection and that of their patients.

17.2   Where relevant locally or nationally agreed guidelines exist for the diagnosis and management of the condition, these should be consulted as part of the clinical assessment. Additional advice should be sought where necessary.

Presently there is a limited number of conditions for which guidelines are available[54] but the BMA would like to see more developed. Where guidelines are not available and there is reasonable doubt about the diagnosis or prognosis or where the health care team has limited experience of the condition, particularly with comparatively rare disorders, advice should be sought from another senior clinician with experience of the condition before making decisions about withdrawing or withholding life-prolonging treatment. Where, for example, assessments are required about the extent of brain damage and the likelihood of any degree of recovery, advice will usually be required from a clinician with expertise in the long-term consequences and management of brain injury.

Existing resources should be utilised where additional advice is needed. Professional bodies, such as the BMA and the Royal Colleges, defence bodies, Trust solicitors, the Office of the Official Solicitor (in England, Wales and Northern Ireland) and the Scottish Office Solicitors (in Scotland) are all able to provide general advice in individual cases if necessary.

In case of challenge or disagreement, health professionals must be able to demonstrate a reasonable justification for their decisions including those which deviate from established guidance. Detailed notes should be kept of any guidelines consulted or additional opinions sought.

17.3 Where treatment is unable to achieve its intended clinical goal or the patient's imminent death is inevitable, active treatment may provide no benefit and may be withheld or withdrawn.

Whilst active treatment may be stopped in these circumstances (including artificial nutrition and hydration), basic care should always be provided (including the offer of oral nutrition and hydration and any procedure necessary to keep the patient comfortable). Efforts should be made to make the patient's life and environment as positive and as comfortable as possible. The basis on which the decision to withdraw or withhold treatment was made, and subsequent action, should be recorded in the medical notes.

17.4 Except where the patient's imminent death is inevitable, a decision to withhold or withdraw *all* treatment is likely to be inappropriate and potentially unlawful. Assessments should be based on whether each potentially available treatment would benefit the patient, taking account of the residual effect of any remaining medication or treatment on the patient.

An important part of the assessment will include consideration of the effect of continuing to provide some treatment in isolation from the medical procedure being withdrawn. Where ventilatory support is to be withdrawn, for example, consideration must be given to the continuing residual effect of any medication which has been provided which has the effect of suppressing the patient's ability to breathe unaided. Failure to do so could be interpreted, in law, as action taken with the purpose or objective of ending the patient's life (see section 19.1).

17.5 Where the patient has an existing condition which means that the progression of the disorder is known or it is recognised that cardiac arrest is likely, consideration should be given in advance to formulating a management plan to anticipate such events. Such plans, and the reasons for them, should be recorded in the medical notes.

Advance planning for anticipated medical events or the progression of the disorder allows more time for discussion with the patient, if he or she has sufficient capacity, those close to the patient if the patient lacks capacity and for discussion and reflection within the health care team. This avoids the need to make decisions abruptly. One common example of advance planning concerns decisions relating to cardiopulmonary resuscitation.[55]

17.6 Where a patient presents with a sudden or unexpected medical event, there is likely to be initial uncertainty about the diagnosis, the likely effectiveness of treatment and the long-term prognosis. In these cases, the initial efforts should be focused on stabilising the patient, so that a proper assessment of the condition

may be undertaken and the likelihood and extent of any expected improvement can be assessed.

In the immediate aftermath of an accident, injury, stroke or onset of an unexpected condition, the initial efforts will be aimed at stabilising the patient's condition to allow time for a proper assessment. Time is an important factor in relation to recovery rates for many medical conditions and questions about the continuation or initiation of treatment are more likely to arise when patients fail to demonstrate any improvement over a prolonged period.

17.7 Where there is reasonable doubt about its potential for benefit, treatment should be provided for a trial period with a subsequent prearranged review. If, following the review, it is decided that the treatment has failed or ceased to be of benefit to the patient, consideration should be given to its withdrawal.

Where insufficient information is available about the severity of the condition or the likelihood of recovery at the time a decision is needed, treatment should be provided although this may be for a trial period with a prearranged review. With stroke patients, for example, where the outcome is uncertain, all appropriate treatment, including artificial nutrition and hydration, should usually be provided in order to stabilise the patient to give time for proper assessment. The treatment may, however, be withdrawn following a review, after a predetermined period, if it is considered that the patient's condition is so severe that the burdens of providing the treatment outweigh the benefits. Where the treatment to be withdrawn is artificial nutrition and hydration, the BMA recommends that additional safeguards should be followed (see Part 3D).

Where treatment is provided for a trial period, this should be made unambiguously clear at the outset to all those involved in the care of the patient including, where appropriate, the relatives or those close to the patient and, where appointed, a health care proxy. A decision should be made, in advance, about when the review will take place and the factors which will be taken into account in deciding whether to continue to provide treatment after the review.

In emergency situations where there is doubt about the

appropriateness of treatment and no prior decision has been made, there should be a presumption in favour of providing life-prolonging treatment even though this may be withdrawn at a later stage when more information is available.

17.8 Before a decision is made to withhold or withdraw treatment, adequate time, resources and facilities should be made available to permit a thorough assessment of the patient's condition including, where appropriate, the patient's potential for self-awareness, awareness of others and the ability intentionally to interact with them. This should involve a multidisciplinary team with expertise in undertaking this type of assessment.

Once the patient's condition has stabilised and an accurate assessment of the condition and prognosis has been made, the decision to provide life-prolonging treatment should be reappraised to ensure that it continues to provide a benefit to the patient. Where the patient is in a stable but profoundly impaired condition, with no prospect of any reasonable degree of improvement, and appears to be unable to communicate in any meaningful way, further investigations may be needed to assess factors such as the patient's level of self-awareness, awareness of others and the ability intentionally to interact with them. This is a specialised task and very great care is needed to ensure that this assessment has been thoroughly undertaken by professionals with expertise in an appropriate range of assessment techniques. For example, an experienced psychologist and speech therapist may be able to provide additional insights to those of the usual treating team. Steps should be taken to optimise the conditions for such assessments such as ensuring that the patient is well nourished, that the use of sedatives is kept to a minimum and that the patient's physical environment is conducive to the best possible assessment of his or her capabilities. Adequate time should be set aside for the assessment which should, ideally, be undertaken over a period by an experienced multidisciplinary team. Decision making should be transparent and able to withstand close scrutiny.

17.9 Treatment should never be withheld merely on the grounds that it is more convenient or easier to withhold treatment than to withdraw treatment which has been initiated.

Where there is genuine doubt about the ability of a particular treatment to provide a benefit to the patient, it should be provided, even though it may subsequently be withdrawn when more information is available. The duty to protect life in Article 2 of the European Convention can be breached by omissions as well as by actions. It would be unacceptable to withhold any treatment, including artificial nutrition and hydration, on the grounds that it is considered easier (for example, for the family to accept) to withhold the treatment than to withdraw that which has already been started. Similarly, a non-beneficial treatment should not be provided for the sake of the family.

17.10 The benefits, risks and burdens of the treatment in the particular case should be assessed.

Where the treatment would achieve its intended clinical aim but the chances of recovery, or the level of recovery which can reasonably be expected, are very small, consideration should be given to whether the risks and harms of treatment outweigh the benefits for the individual patient. Wherever available, evidence-based data should be used for comparing benefits and burdens.

Evaluation must be undertaken on a case-by-case basis rather than assuming that the same treatment decisions will be appropriate for all patients with a particular condition. Sometimes, a balance between benefit and harm cannot be confidently predicted. In each clinical circumstance the doctor must make a careful and conscientious judgment, recognising the elusiveness of certainty regarding the consequences of the decision. This judgment must take account of all relevant medical, ethical and legal considerations and best established practice in that area.

17.11 All treatment decisions should be reviewed on a regular basis both before and after implementation.

Regular review should be undertaken by the clinician in charge of the patient's care in consultation with the rest of the health care team to take account of any changing circumstances before or after implementation of the decision. Decisions should also be subject to audit to ensure that appropriate procedures were followed and that the decisions were properly documented.

17.12 With the exception of those patients whose imminent death is inevitable or whose wishes are known, decisions to withhold or withdraw artificial nutrition and hydration should be subject to additional safeguards (see Part 3D).

18.   Ethical factors to be considered

18.1 Both legally and ethically, treatment provided for a person who is unable to consent for him or herself must promote that individual's best interests.

Best interests presents an apparently reassuring standard by which decisions should be made but can be interpreted in many ways. In the past, best interests were often seen solely in terms of best medical interests and the prolongation of life at almost any cost was often regarded as being in the patient's interests. Modern technology and the ability to sustain some essential functions far beyond the irrevocable loss of awareness and ability to interact with others increasingly demonstrate this to be unsustainable. Legal judgments about the withdrawal of life-prolonging treatment have now made clear that, in some circumstances, invasive prolongation of life need not be provided either because it can be perceived as a harm or would not provide a health benefit to that individual.

In each case of patients in persistent vegetative state (pvs) that the law has considered, it has decided that it would not be unlawful to withdraw artificial nutrition and hydration, on the basis that its provision was not in the best interests of the individual patient. (By the end of September 2000, 23 such cases had been considered by the courts and two were heard in early October 2000 in which the court confirmed that withdrawing or withholding artificial nutrition and hydration in such circumstances did not contravene the Human Rights Act, see section 19.1.) Some legal commentators have suggested that the inevitable conclusion to be reached from these cases is that artificial nutrition and hydration would never be in the best interests of a patient in pvs and should always be withdrawn. As stressed throughout this document, however, the BMA believes that such important decisions must only be made after very careful consideration of the individual circumstances in each case, rather than applying blanket decisions to certain categories of patients.

Patients in pvs have a permanent and irreversible lack of awareness of themselves or their surroundings and no ability to interact at any level with those around them. Other patients, who are not in pvs but have very severe brain damage, have some, but very limited, levels of awareness. Two people with the same level of awareness may, but do not necessarily, have the same best interests. Decisions should be made on the basis of what is right for each individual patient. The type of factors which should be taken into account in assessing whether the provision of life-prolonging treatment would provide an overall health benefit to the patient include:

- the patient's own wishes and values (where these can be ascertained);
- clinical judgment about the effectiveness of the proposed treatment;
- the likelihood of the patient experiencing severe unmanageable pain or suffering;
- the level of awareness the individual has of his or her existence and surroundings as demonstrated by, for example:
  - an ability to interact with others, however expressed;
  - capacity for self-directed action or ability to take control of any aspect of his or her life;
- the likelihood and extent of any degree of improvement in the patient's condition if treatment is provided;
- whether the invasiveness of the treatment is justified in the circumstances;
- the views of the parents, if the patient is a child;
- the views of people close to the patient, especially close relatives, partners and carers, about what the patient is likely to see as beneficial;

• in Scotland; the views of an appointed health care proxy.

Taking account of these and any other relevant factors, decisions must be made in each case which can be justified in terms of the benefit to the individual patient.

18.2 Although ultimately the responsibility for treatment decisions rests with the clinician in charge of the patient's care, it is important, where non-emergency decisions are made, that account is taken of the views of other health professionals involved in the patient's care and people close to the patient, in order to ensure that the decision is as well informed as possible. In Scotland, certain other people will have a legal right to be consulted under the Adults with Incapacity (Scotland) Act (see section 13.4).

The importance of team working in providing health care is widely recognised and is particularly important when making complex decisions about whether to withhold or withdraw life-prolonging treatment. Seeking agreement within the team about the most appropriate course of action can help to reduce the possibility of subjectivity or bias in cases of uncertainty. All health professionals involved with caring for the patient have an important contribution to make to the assessment; nurses often have a particular insight into the patient's wishes and may have spent considerable time with the patient and the patient's relatives. Many nurses have reported concern about what they perceive as "moral distancing" on the part of some doctors. They consider that those who make the decision generally delegate its implementation to nurses, who can feel unhappy if they have not been able to contribute in any way to that decision. Depending upon the type of treatment under consideration, it may be appropriate to involve a dietician, speech therapist, psychologist, physiotherapist and other members of the team who have been involved in the patient's care. The patient's general practitioner is often able to provide valuable information about the patient's wishes or values. The patient's general practice notes may include discussions with the patient about future treatment, particularly if the patient was aware that he or she was suffering from a progressive illness in the period before decision making capacity, or the ability to communicate, was lost.

18.3 Even where their views have no legal status in terms of actual decision making, those close to the patient may have a right to be consulted. In any event it is clear that they can provide important information to help ascertain whether the patient would have considered life-prolonging treatment to be beneficial.

The views of people close to an adult patient carry no legal weight, although in Scotland there may be an appointed proxy decision maker (see section 13.4) and those with parental responsibility have the legal authority to make most decisions for children (see Part 3B). The Human Rights Act may also lead to rights to consultation with respect to treatment decisions. Even where they do not have legal authority, however, the views of those close to an adult patient can be of considerable value in helping to clarify what the patient would have considered to be beneficial and so should generally be consulted. In addition in Scotland, the Adults with Incapacity (Scotland) Act provides a legal obligation to take account of the views of the nearest relatives and primary carer of an incapacitated adult patient. It is important to be clear, however, that the information sought relates to any views the patient expressed when competent which might help to ascertain what he or she would have wanted in these circumstances, as opposed to what those consulted would like for the patient or what they would want for themselves if they were in the same situation. In practice, the extent to which friends and relatives are able to inform the doctor's decision is likely to be dependent upon whether the patient has discussed the issues with them. Knowing the patient, however, they may be able to give a clearer picture of the type of values the patient held and the things which were important to the patient when competent.

Although important, seeking views from those close to a patient who has lost decision making capacity, or the ability to communicate, is not unproblematic. Studies have shown that relatives' perceptions of the patient's likely views often differ substantially from the patient's own wishes.[56] Often, relatives tend to have a more negative impression of the condition than the patient him or herself but, on the other hand, they may not wish to see themselves as responsible for the withholding of treatment and so insist the patient would want treatment to continue. There is also a risk that an "off the cuff" remark, made without careful consideration of the implications, may be given inappropriate significance and taken as evidence of the individual's wishes. Particular difficulties can arise where there is disagreement within the family about what the patient would have wanted or where conflicting information is given by relatives. Concern may also arise where the family may be thought to have motives other than the patient's best interests. Recognising these difficulties, however, seeking information from those close to the patient presents the only opportunity for the health team to gain any impression of the patient's likely wishes and values. Information should be sought, wherever possible, from more than one person and great care is needed in interpreting any information received which should be seen as one part of a wider decision making process rather than necessarily being judged as conclusive. The final decision must be that which promotes the best interests of the incompetent patient and relatives and carers may need varying degrees of support to come to terms with the decision.

Health professionals are well aware that discussion with those close to the patient about withholding or withdrawing life-prolonging treatment needs sensitive handling. Time and thought need to be given to how partners, parents and relatives can discuss the diagnosis, prognosis and treatment options in an unpressured environment. It can sometimes be helpful to formalise such discussions, as in a case conference, to include the main members of the health care team and the people closest to the patient although some relatives find such meetings intimidating.

In talking to those close to the patient a balance must be sought between preserving confidentiality and obtaining sufficient information to make an informed assessment. Where a patient has, when competent, expressed a specific wish that his or her condition should not be discussed with relatives or friends, this should be respected, not least because after the Human Rights Act, the patient is entitled to respect for his or her privacy under Article 8 of the European Convention.[57] This should not, however, prevent the health care team from seeking information from them about the patient's wishes and values. In addition to seeking information to take into account in assessing whether treatment would provide a benefit to the patient, discussing the issues with those close to the patient (where this would not be contrary to the patient's expressed wishes) can also be helpful in helping them to come to terms with the situation. It may be useful, as part of this discussion, to emphasise that the health care team and those close to the patient are all working towards the same aim – to benefit the patient – even if their views as to how that can best be achieved may differ.

Whilst the views of those close to the patient will be an important factor to take into account in reaching treatment decisions, it is essential that those consulted are absolutely clear that, ultimately, the treatment decision is not their right or their responsibility (although the decisions of health care proxies in Scotland will carry some legal weight (see section 13.4)). The decision will be made by the clinician in charge of the patient's care on the basis of what he or she considers will benefit the patient.

18.4 Good communication, both within the health care team and between the health team and the patient and/or those close to the patient, is an essential part of decision making. Wherever possible, consensus should be sought amongst all those consulted about whether the provision of life-prolonging treatment would benefit the patient.

A lack of consensus in decision making frequently results from poor communication and inadequate provision of accurate information to all those involved in the decision. This should include the patient, if he or she has sufficient capacity to understand, and those close to the patient if the patient lacks the capacity to make or communicate a decision. It is important that all those involved in the decision understand why it has been made, on what grounds and with what implications. Doctors not only have an obligation to ensure that the most reliable and accurate data are used to make the decision but also to ensure that those data can be accessed by everyone closely involved in the decision, including relatives of an incompetent adult where this can be achieved without disclosing information the patient wished to remain confidential. Where information is provided to those close to the patient, this should be done sensitively and efforts should be made to provide the information in a way which can be easily understood by those who do not have medical training or a detailed knowledge of the condition.

Conflict within the clinical team is likely to undermine the confidence of relatives that the right decision is being made. Hospital managers have an obligation to ensure that conflict management strategies are in place, such as an external mediator, and that junior medical and nursing staff, as well as carers and people close to the patient, can express informally any misgivings they have about the basis of the decisions made. Patients and relatives already have a formal complaints procedure but some of their concerns may be resolvable by informal discussion. It is also important that nurses and other staff can air their views within the team without fear that it will jeopardise their career prospects. (See also section 24 on conscientious objection.)

Where there is serious conflict within the health care team or between the health care team and those close to the patient, attempts should be made to resolve this through discussion, informal conflict resolution mechanisms or by obtaining a further independent opinion. General advice may be sought from the Official Solicitor, in England, Wales and Northern Ireland, or the Scottish Office Solicitors in Scotland. In rare cases, consideration may need to be given to seeking a legal review of the decision before its implementation.

18.5 Patients who have lost or never attained competence, including babies, are entitled to the same quality of care as other patients and should not be excluded from potentially beneficial, but costly, treatment options solely by reason of their incapacity.

Existing guidelines and court judgments have insisted that non-treatment decisions for people who lack the ability to make or communicate decisions should be based on considerations of benefit to the patient and not cost. It is obvious, however, that money spent caring for irreversibly and severely brain-damaged patients is money which cannot be used to treat other patients. This is an issue which needs to be acknowledged and addressed on

57

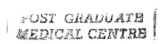

a national scale as part of the debate on rationing and prioritising of resources. The BMA is concerned that, in reality, cost factors probably have a disproportionate influence on decision making for this very vulnerable patient group and is also concerned that the lack of a clear societal consensus on this most vexed area may unfairly leave doctors open to criticism. Doctors must be able to show that all materially relevant criteria have been considered for those with and without mental incapacity, in deciding whether to offer treatment. The issue is likely to become very prominent in view of the legal obligation placed on all public authorities not to discriminate unjustifiably in the protection of the rights of patients (see in particular Articles 2 and 14 of the European Convention).

19. Legal factors to be considered

19.1 Although the health care team may foresee that withholding or withdrawing life-prolonging treatment will result in the patient's death, this is fundamentally different from action taken with the purpose or objective of ending the patient's life.

Some people have argued that a doctor deciding to withhold or withdraw life-prolonging treatment (including, but not only, artificial nutrition and hydration) which will inevitably or very probably result in the patient's death *must* be doing so with the purpose or objective of ending that person's life. The BMA does not share this view. A doctor may withhold or withdraw life-prolonging treatment if the purpose of doing so is to withdraw treatment which is not a benefit to the patient and is therefore not in the patient's best interests.

In law, a doctor may foresee – be able to predict – that the patient will die if treatment is not provided but this *cannot* be the sole reason for withholding it; the *overriding* purpose or objective is to ensure that treatment which is not in the best interests of the patient is avoided.[58] It is only when this condition is satisfied that withholding or withdrawing treatment without the patient's consent will be lawful. In other words, it is only lawful to withhold or withdraw treatment when to continue it is not in the patient's best interests. The courts have confirmed that, in such circumstances, the health team would not be in breach of its duty to protect life under Article 2 of the European Convention. Just days after the implementation of the Human Rights Act, the High Court authorised the withdrawal of artificial nutrition and hydration from two patients in a persistent vegetative state (pvs).[59] The court confirmed that where withdrawing or withholding artificial nutrition and hydration is in a patient's best interests, there is no breach of Article 2.

19.2 BMA policy "recognises that there is a wide spectrum of views about the issues of physician-assisted suicide and euthanasia and strongly opposes any changes in law for the time being".[60]

19.3 Decisions to withhold or withdraw conventional treatment, on the basis that it is not providing a benefit to the patient, should be made by the clinician in overall charge of the patient's care following discussion with the rest of the health care team and, where appropriate, those close to the patient and any appointed health care proxy. Where the clinician's view is seriously challenged and agreement cannot be reached by other means, review by a court would be advisable. Decisions to withhold or withdraw artificial nutrition and hydration from patients whose imminent death is not inevitable, and whose wishes are not known, require additional safeguards which are discussed in Part 3D.

As discussed in section 13.3, the case of *Re F*[61] established that treatment may be provided to an incompetent adult but in order for the treatment to be lawful, there must be some necessity to act when it is not practicable to communicate with the assisted person and the action taken must be in that person's best interests. A similar principle is enshrined in the Adults with Incapacity (Scotland) Act which gives doctors the authority to do what is reasonable in the circumstances to safeguard or promote an incapacitated patient's physical or mental health where no proxy has been appointed. Where the treatment is not necessary (ie "action properly taken to preserve the life, health or well-being of the assisted person") and in the best interests of the patient there is no authority for providing the treatment and, in fact, to provide treatment could be considered an assault or battery. Thus, the law states that incompetent adults should not be subjected to procedures or treatments which are of no benefit to them.

Further guidance about the scope and process of decision making was provided in the 1996 case of *Re R*.[62] R was 23 years old and had been born with a serious malformation of the brain and cerebral palsy. He also developed severe epilepsy, had profound learning disability and had not developed any formal means of communication or any consistent interactions with his social environment. He was unable to walk, was believed to be blind and deaf and had a range of other health problems. In the expert clinical evidence provided, it was stated that R was believed to be operating cognitively and neurologically at the level of a newborn infant.

The health care team and the parents were in agreement that should R have a further life-threatening crisis, cardiopulmonary resuscitation or antibiotics should not be provided as such treatment would not provide a benefit to him. This assessment of R's best interests was challenged by a third party and so the High Court was asked to consider the case. The challenge was made on the basis that the decision was "irrational and unlawful in that [the decisions to withhold cardiopulmonary resuscitation and antibiotics] permit medical treatment to be withheld on the basis of an assessment of a patient's quality of life". The court dismissed the appeal. It made clear, however, that decisions should be made on the basis of whether a particular treatment would confer a benefit on the patient – taking account of both medical factors and whether the treatment was able to provide a reasonable quality of life for the patient – rather than a blanket decision to provide no treatment.

In that case, the High Court clarified that "the decision as to the withholding of the administration of antibiotics in a potentially life-threatening situation is a matter fully within the responsibility of the consultant having the responsibility for treating the patient". Drawing on the 1990 case of *Re J* (see section 14.2), the court stated that the overriding principle, in considering whether treatment would be in the patient's best interests, was the same for an incompetent adult as for a child and consideration should be given to whether the patient's life, if treatment were given, would be "so afflicted as to be intolerable". Such cases have always been difficult and, under the Human Rights Act, doctors must balance the duty to protect life on the one hand and the duty not to cause inhuman or degrading treatment on the other.

The judgment in the *Re R* case referred specifically to the provision of antibiotics for life-threatening infection and cardiopulmonary resuscitation. This case needs to be considered, however, in conjunction with other judgments, such as the general guidance in *Re F* about when the provision of treatment is justified (see above) and the statement made in the 1992 case of *Re J* [63] that Lord Justice Leggatt, echoing Lord Donaldson and Lord Justice Balcombe, could "envisage no circumstances in which it would be right directly or indirectly to require a doctor to treat a patient in a way that was contrary to the doctor's professional judgment and duty to the patient". It is clear from these cases that the appropriate person to make decisions about whether to provide treatment for an incompetent adult is the clinician in charge of the patient's care, provided that the decision is reasonable in the light of all relevant factors.

Given that, as discussed in section 3.4, artificial nutrition and hydration has been classified by the courts as medical treatment, it might be assumed that the same criteria would apply as for other, more conventional, forms of treatment. The House of Lords, however, indicated that additional safeguards should be in place for the withdrawal of artificial nutrition and hydration from patients in persistent vegetative state (by recommending that all such cases within its jurisdiction should, for the time being, be referred to the courts). The same requirement has not been made in relation to the withdrawal of artificial nutrition and hydration from patients in other conditions, or for patients in persistent vegetative state in Scotland. The BMA believes that wherever artificial nutrition and hydration is to be withdrawn from patients whose imminent death is not inevitable and whose wishes are not known, additional safeguards should be in place (see Part 3D). The BMA is concerned that the provision of judicial safeguards for certain patients for whom withdrawal or withholding of life-prolonging treatment is being considered, and not for others in a similar situation, may violate Article 14 of the European Convention. If the courts were to remove the requirement for court review for patients in persistent vegetative state, as discussed in sections 21.1 and 21.4, this could avoid a potential breach of Article 14.

19.4 Where professional guidance is available which represents the views of a responsible body of medical opinion, this may be used by doctors and the courts to determine the acceptability of a particular practice.

In many legal cases concerning treatment, judges rely on professional medical guidance or codes of practice in reaching decisions. Professional guidance, which represents the views of a responsible body of medical opinion, can provide important information and advice about good practice and may be adopted by the courts in a particular case although it does not, in itself, have legal standing. Whilst professional guidance cannot be followed blindly, if it has a logical basis and is factually correct, a doctor acting in accordance with the guidance in a particular case is likely to be seen to have acted reasonably.

PART 3D   Decisions about withholding or withdrawing artificial nutrition and hydration

20.   Additional guidance

20.1 The guidance set out in Part 3C applies to all decisions to withhold or withdraw life-prolonging treatment. Where the decision relates to artificial nutrition and hydration, however, the additional factors discussed in this section also need to be considered.

Although the BMA welcomes the categorisation of artificial nutrition and hydration as a form of medical treatment, it accepts that many people perceive there to be an important distinction between this and other treatments. In recognition of this fact and in order to reassure patients, their families and society as a whole that decisions to withhold or withdraw artificial nutrition and hydration are taken only in the most extreme cases, where its provision would not provide a net benefit to the patient, it is recommended that additional procedural safeguards should be followed. Additional procedural safeguards are proposed in section 22.

21. Legal considerations

21.1 In England, Wales and Northern Ireland, proposals to withdraw artificial nutrition and hydration from a patient who is in persistent vegetative state, or in a state of very low awareness closely resembling pvs, currently require legal review.

In 1993, the House of Lords concluded that it would not be unlawful to withdraw artificial nutrition and hydration from a patient, Tony Bland, who was in persistent vegetative state. This was based on the view that artificial nutrition and hydration constituted medical treatment, the continued provision of which was not in his best interests. It was acknowledged at the time, however, that Bland's condition was very extreme and that in other cases where such action was proposed, the assessment of best interests may be less clear. In view of this and the very emotive nature of the withdrawal of artificial nutrition and hydration, the House of Lords recommended that, for the time being, in all cases where the withdrawal of artificial nutrition and hydration was being considered from a patient in pvs, a court declaration should be sought. It was clearly stated that this should be an interim measure until a body of experience had developed and other effective mechanisms for decision making had been put in place. As expertise and professional guidelines develop on persistent vegetative state, the BMA can see no reason to differentiate between decisions for patients in pvs and those for patients with other serious conditions where artificial nutrition and hydration is not considered to be a benefit, which are currently governed by established practice without the need for legal review. The BMA hopes that in future the courts will decide that pvs cases no longer inevitably require court review, where consensus exists, as long as such withdrawal is in accordance with agreed guidance. The BMA believes that such a change would have the added advantage of the removal of a possible discriminatory practice contra to Article 14 of the European Convention (see section 19.3).

Presently, however, the clear advice from the English courts is that a declaration should be sought for each case in which it is proposed to withdraw artificial nutrition and hydration from a patient in pvs or a condition closely resembling pvs. (Since the current guidance states that the patient must have been in the condition for at least six months before a diagnosis of pvs can be confirmed, the question of *withholding* artificial nutrition and hydration from patients in this condition does not arise.) Whilst this advice is helpful in guiding and providing a degree of legal protection for health professionals, the legal effectiveness of such declarations has been questioned. A declaration from the court cannot make lawful a procedure which would otherwise be unlawful. If the action is lawful with the declaration, it would also be lawful without the declaration. The advantage of seeking such a declaration, however, is to assess, before the treatment is withdrawn, whether this action is considered to be reasonable in the particular case and to provide reassurance that all relevant factors have been considered. The withdrawal of artificial nutrition and hydration from a patient who is in pvs without a court declaration may be lawful but it would at present leave the doctor open to criticism, and potentially legal challenge, for failing to follow established procedures and guidelines.

21.2 In Scotland the withdrawal of artificial nutrition and hydration from a patient in pvs does not require a court declaration.

A Scottish court has also authorised the withdrawal of artificial nutrition and hydration from a patient in pvs.[64] Unlike in England, the judgment made it explicitly clear that it was not necessary to apply to the courts in every case where the withdrawal of artificial nutrition and hydration is proposed from a patient in pvs. The court of Session has confirmed its authority to consider such cases but did not make such consideration a formal requirement. The Lord Advocate further indicated that, where such authority has been granted by the Court of Session, the doctor would not face prosecution. This leaves open the possibility of prosecution should the doctor not seek authority from the Court of Session.

In Scotland general advice may be sought from the Scottish Office Solicitors and, although a court declaration may not be necessary, some doctors or hospitals may prefer to seek this reassurance.

21.3 Where the patient's imminent death is believed to be inevitable, artificial nutrition and hydration may be withheld or withdrawn if it is not considered to be a benefit to the patient.

Once an individual's condition has reached the stage where death is imminent, such as in the final stages of a terminal illness, the focus of care changes from attempting to prolong life to keeping the patient as comfortable as possible until death occurs. In these final stages, active treatment and the provision of artificial nutrition and hydration may become unnecessarily intrusive and merely prolong the dying process rather than offering a benefit to the patient. Basic care should, however, always be provided (including the offer of oral nutrition and hydration and any procedure necessary to keep the patient comfortable).

In England, Wales and Northern Ireland the authority to treat incapacitated adults was articulated in the House of Lords' decision in *Re F* (see section 13.3), which made clear that treatment may only be provided for an incompetent adult where this would be necessary and in the best interests of the patient. In Scotland, the Adults with Incapacity (Scotland) Act gives doctors the authority to do what is reasonable in the circumstances to safeguard or promote an incapacitated patient's physical or mental health where no proxy has been appointed.

Where death is believed to be imminent and unavoidable, treatment would not be reasonable in order to safeguard the patient's health, and could in fact be contrary to his or her best interests by providing the burden of the treatment without any benefit. Although, as stated in section 3.4, the courts have distinguished between withholding or withdrawing conventional treatment and artificial nutrition and hydration, in terms of its withholding or withdrawing, in this situation the patient would be expected to die of his or her condition before the effect of ceasing nutrition and hydration was operative.

21.4 The courts have not specified that declarations should be sought before withholding or withdrawing

artificial nutrition and hydration from patients who are not in persistent vegetative state. Although a body of medical opinion has developed that such action would be appropriate in some cases (such as some patients who have suffered a serious stroke or have severe dementia), United Kingdom courts have not yet considered such a case. This arguably leaves doctors in an area of legal uncertainty and therefore open to challenge particularly following implementation of the Human Rights Act (see section 19.3). Particular care needs to be taken when making such decisions and the BMA believes that additional safeguards should be followed (see section 22).

Decisions about artificial nutrition and hydration sometimes arise in connection with common conditions which currently are not taken to court but around which a body of practice has evolved. Such cases arise, for example, when elderly patients suffer from profound and irreversible dementia or have suffered a stroke which has left them similarly irreversibly brain damaged. An assessment must be made of whether the provision of artificial nutrition and hydration would provide a net benefit to the patient, taking account of the burdens of the treatment[65] and the possibility of any improvement in the patient's condition. Existing guidance from the courts on the withdrawal of artificial nutrition and hydration refers only to patients in persistent vegetative state and United Kingdom courts have not yet considered other cases. Clearly this situation may change over time. If, subsequent to the publication of this guidance, authoritative legal rulings are made, doctors must respect them.[66] Subject to any such rulings, and in the absence of any serious conflict of opinion or uncertainty about the patient's prognosis, however, the BMA does not consider that all such decisions require legal review and no medical or legal body has suggested that legal review of routine practice in this area would be helpful. Indeed, given the number of patients suffering from these conditions, such a suggestion is likely to be logistically impossible to implement. Doctors should, however, be aware that until the courts have specifically considered a case of this type, their discretion to make decisions to withdraw artificial nutrition and hydration in these circumstances could be challenged. This lack of clarity is unsatisfactory for health professionals, patients and their relatives and it is hoped that the law will be clarified in the near future.

22. Additional procedural safeguards

22.1 The BMA believes that, in addition to the guidance in Part 3C, the following additional safeguards should be applied to decisions to withhold or withdraw artificial nutrition and hydration from patients whose death is not imminent and whose wishes are not known.

The withholding or withdrawing of artificial nutrition and hydration will inevitably result in the patient's death. This is also true of some other treatments, such as the provision of insulin for an insulin-dependent diabetic, and there are arguments for applying the same procedural safeguards to some other forms of treatment. This is a matter for individual doctors, and those developing local policies and guidelines, to consider.

(a) All proposals to withhold or withdraw artificial nutrition and hydration whether in hospital or in the community should be subject to formal clinical review by a senior clinician who has experience of the condition from which the patient is suffering and who is not part of the treating team.

The level of specialisation required to undertake the clinical review will depend upon the condition and for rarer conditions, this may involve seeking advice from an expert from a particular specialty or a doctor specialising in the long-term care of patients with severe brain injury or in persistent vegetative state. For more common conditions, the senior clinician could be a general practitioner, particularly where the patient is being treated in the community, such as in a nursing home.

The clinical review should involve this senior clinician reviewing the patient's notes, examining the patient and discussing the circumstances with the treating doctor. The views of this person should be recorded in the medical record.

(b) In England, Wales and Northern Ireland, where it is proposed to withdraw artificial nutrition and

hydration from a patient in persistent vegetative state or a state closely resembling pvs, legal advice should be sought and a court declaration is likely to be required until such time as the courts have stated otherwise.

In all cases in England, Wales and Northern Ireland where it is proposed to withdraw artificial nutrition and hydration from a patient in pvs or a condition closely resembling pvs, until such time as the courts decide otherwise, legal advice should be sought. General advice may be sought from the Official Solicitor and a court declaration is likely to be required. It is also advisable for medical teams facing the same situation in Scotland to consider carefully whether similar recourse to the courts should not also be initiated.

(c)   All cases in which artificial nutrition and hydration has been withdrawn should be available for clinical review to ensure that appropriate procedures and guidelines were followed. Anonymised information should also be available to the Secretary of State on request and, where applicable, the Commission for Health Improvement.

Mechanisms should be in place to identify all cases in which artificial nutrition and hydration was withheld or withdrawn from patients who were not imminently dying and where the patients' wishes were not known. These cases should be reviewed, at a local level, in order to ensure that appropriate procedures and guidelines were followed.

The Commission for Health Improvement is designed to provide an independent guarantee that local systems monitor, assure and improve clinical quality. It is also intended to support local development and "spot-check" local arrangements. The BMA recommends that, for the areas it covers, this body also monitor patterns of ethical decision making in controversial areas such as the withdrawal or withholding of artificial nutrition and hydration from patients who lack decision making capacity who are not dying.

PART 4 Once a decision has been reached to withhold or withdraw life-prolonging treatment

23. Informing others of the decision

23.1 Every effort should be made to explain to the patient, to the extent that he or she can understand, the decision which has been reached and the reasons for that decision.

The patient should be encouraged to discuss the decision to withhold or withdraw treatment to the extent that he or she is able and willing to do so.

23.2 Wherever possible, before implementing a decision to withdraw or withhold treatment, those consulted in the process of reaching the decision should be informed of the final decision.

Although there is no obligation to inform those close to the patient (subject to any new obligations that the courts might impose under the Human Rights Act), or the rest of the team, about the basis on which the decision to withhold or withdraw treatment was made, it is good practice to do so. Such an explanation can help those involved with providing care for the patient to satisfy themselves that the proposed treatment would not provide a benefit to the patient and can help those close to the patient to come to terms with the situation. It also gives advance notice of any disagreement about the patient's care which may necessitate further discussion, a further medical opinion or, if the matter cannot be resolved and there is persistent disagreement, a legal review of the case.

24. Conscientious objection

24.1 Where a member of the health care team has a conscientious objection to withholding or withdrawing life-prolonging treatment, he or she should, wherever possible, be permitted to hand over care of the patient to a colleague. This is a best practice which may also now be necessitated by the guarantee of freedom of conscience in Article 9 of the European Convention.

Some people have a fundamental objection to withholding or withdrawing life-prolonging treatment, particularly where the treatment in question is artificial nutrition and hydration. Where there is general agreement that further treatment would not provide a net benefit to the patient and the appropriate safeguards have been followed, any member of the team with a conscientious objection to such withdrawal should, wherever possible, be permitted to hand over his or her role in the care of the patient to a colleague. Where, however, an individual does not disagree in principle with withdrawing or withholding life-prolonging treatment but considers the action to be unjustified in the particular case and can produce reasonable arguments to that effect, further discussion will be required to attempt to resolve this conflict, possibly by seeking a further medical opinion or independent review.

25. Recording and reviewing the decision

25.1 The basis for the decision to withhold or withdraw life-prolonging treatment should be carefully documented in the patient's medical notes.

The clinician in charge of the patient's care should clearly record in the notes when and by whom the decision was made to withhold or withdraw a particular treatment, the basis on which the decision was reached, from whom information was received and the way in which it was used. Where treatment is refused by a competent adult, the patient should be asked to provide written confirmation of the refusal, if possible, and this should be held in the medical record. Where treatment is withheld or withdrawn in response to a valid advance refusal of treatment, a copy of the directive should be held on the record together with a note of any further enquiries made about its validity. If a formal clinical review was undertaken for the withholding or withdrawing of artificial nutrition and hydration, this should be recorded in the medical record as should information about any other professional guidance consulted or advice sought.

Where patients are being cared for by their general practitioner in the community, such as in a nursing home, information should be recorded in both the general practitioner's notes and the nursing or medical notes held within the establishment within which the patient is being cared for.

25.2 Decisions to withhold or withdraw life-prolonging treatment should be reviewed before and after implementation to take account of any change in circumstances.

25.3 Decisions to withdraw or withhold life-prolonging treatment should be subject to review and audit.

Treatment providers and health care facilities have an ethical obligation to audit regularly their own patterns of decision making and compare them with wider trends. Health Authorities should be encouraged to provide local guidelines addressing the decision making process with a system of audit to ensure that the guidelines are being followed. Doctors must be able to demonstrate that their treatment recommendations comply with a responsible body of medical opinion. Advice must be sought from professional bodies and the General Medical Council if anomalous patterns of decision making are identified in comparison with those of other clinicians or other similar facilities. Managers have an obligation to investigate promptly such trends in their facilities.

Those treating patients who lack the capacity to make or communicate decisions need to be aware of the dangers of decisions to withhold or withdraw treatment becoming routinised. A constant awareness is needed that each individual decision must be carefully considered in order to ascertain whether the treatment would provide a net benefit to the particular patient and the doctor must be willing to justify the decision if called upon to do so.

26. Providing support

26.1 Although not responsible for making the decision to withhold or withdraw treatment, those close to the patient are often left with feelings of guilt and anxiety in addition to their bereavement. It is important that the family are supported both before and after the decision has been made to withdraw or withhold life-prolonging treatment.

Providing support for the patient and those close to the patient to help them to come to terms with their bereavement is a routine part of caring for dying patients. Where the patient has died following a decision to withhold or withdraw life-prolonging treatment, however, the usual bereavement may be exacerbated by feelings of guilt or anxiety about whether the right decision was made and about the family's role in that decision. The family should be encouraged to discuss their concerns and, if appropriate, should be offered counselling.

26.2 The emotional and psychological burden on staff involved with withdrawing and withholding life-prolonging treatment should be recognised and adequate support mechanisms need to be available and easily accessible before, during and after decisions have been made.

Staff members' needs for support may easily be overlooked. Employing bodies and colleagues of those involved with making and carrying out these very difficult decisions need to be sensitive to the possibility of "burnout" and to the need for adequate support mechanisms to be in place which are easily accessible to all staff. Staff at all levels should have access to counselling and support both within and outside the health care team. This is likely to be needed before, during and after the decision has been made and implemented.

PART 5   Main points arising from this guidance

This part of the guidance is not designed to be read in isolation from the rest of the document. Given the very serious nature of the decisions being made, we would urge all readers to take the time to consider the whole of the document. This part is intended to highlight some of the main points arising from the guidance, as an *aide-mémoire*.

PART 1 – Setting the scene for decision making

1. The primary goal of medical treatment is to benefit the patient by restoring or maintaining the patient's health as far as possible, maximising benefit and minimising harm. [Section 1.1]

2. If treatment fails, or ceases, to give a net benefit to the patient (or if the patient has competently refused the treatment), the primary goal of medical treatment cannot be realised and the justification for providing the treatment is removed. Unless some other justification can be demonstrated, treatment that does not provide net benefit to the patient may, ethically and legally, be withheld or withdrawn and the goal of medicine should shift to the palliation of symptoms. [Section 1.1]

3. Prolonging a patient's life usually, but not always, provides a health benefit to that patient. It is not an appropriate goal of medicine to prolong life at all costs, with no regard to its quality or the burdens of treatment. [Section 1.2]

4. Although emotionally it may be easier to withhold treatment than to withdraw that which has been started, there are no legal, or necessary morally relevant, differences between the two actions. [Section 6.1]

5. Treatment should never be withheld, when there is a possibility that it will benefit the patient, simply because withholding is considered to be easier than withdrawing treatment. [Section 6.2]

PART 2 – Decisions involving adults who have the capacity to make and communicate decisions or those who have a valid advance directive

6. A voluntary refusal of life-prolonging treatment by a competent adult must be respected. [Section 9.1]
7. Where a patient has lost the capacity to make a decision but has a valid advance directive refusing life-prolonging treatment, this must be respected. [Section 10.1]
8. A valid advance refusal of treatment has the same legal authority as a contemporaneous refusal and legal action could be taken against a doctor who provides treatment in the face of a valid refusal. [Section 10.3]

PART 3 – Decisions involving adults who do not have the capacity to make or communicate decisions and do not have a valid advance directive and decisions involving children and young people

Adults

9. People have varying levels of capacity and should be encouraged to participate in discussion and decision making about all aspects of their lives to the greatest extent possible. The graver the consequences of the decision, the commensurately greater the level of competence required to take that decision. [Section 13.2]
10. At present, in England, Wales and Northern Ireland no other individual has the power to give or withhold consent for the treatment of an adult who lacks decision making capacity but treatment may be provided, without consent, if it is considered by the clinician in charge of the patient's care to be necessary and in the best interests of the patient. [Section 13.3]
11. In Scotland a proxy decision maker may be appointed to give consent to medical treatment on behalf of an incapacitated person over 16 years of age. [Section 13.4]
12. The same principles apply when decisions are taken in relation to a woman who is pregnant with a viable fetus and is unable to make or communicate decisions. Traditionally under UK law the fetus has no legal status and the decision

must be that which represents the best interests of the pregnant woman. The extent to which the woman's likely wishes about the outcome of the pregnancy may be taken into account in determining her best interests is unclear. In order that these matters may be fully explored, legal advice should be sought. In particular it remains to be clarified whether the fetus has Convention rights (in particular the right to life (Article 2) and the right not to be discriminated against (Article 14)) which would be required to be balanced against those of the mother. [Sections 9.4 and 13.7]

Babies, children and young people

13. The same moral duties are owed to babies, children and young people as to adults. [Section 14.1]

14. Those with parental responsibility for a baby or young child are legally and morally entitled to give or withhold consent to treatment. Their decisions will usually be determinative unless they conflict seriously with the interpretation of those providing care about the child's best interests. [Section 15.1]

15. Treatment in a young person's best interests may proceed where there is consent from somebody authorised to give it: the competent young person him or herself, somebody with parental responsibility or a court. It is unclear whether a young person's refusal can, in law, take precedence over the consent of either parents or a court. [Section 16.2]

16. Even where they are not determinative, the views and wishes of competent young people are an essential component of the assessment of their best interests and should, therefore, be given serious consideration at all stages of decision making. [Section 16.3]

The process of decision making

17. Where relevant locally or nationally agreed guidelines exist for the diagnosis and management of the condition, these should be consulted as part of the clinical assessment. Additional advice should be sought where necessary. [Section 17.2]

18. Where there is reasonable doubt about its potential for benefit, treatment should be provided for a trial period with a subsequent prearranged review. If, following the review, it

is decided that the treatment has failed or ceased to be of benefit to the patient, consideration should be given to its withdrawal. [Section 17.7]

19. Before a decision is made to withhold or withdraw treatment, adequate time, resources and facilities should be made available to permit a thorough assessment of the patient's condition including, where appropriate, the patient's potential for self-awareness, awareness of others and the ability intentionally to interact with them. This should involve a multidisciplinary team with expertise in undertaking this type of assessment. [Section 17.8]

20. The benefits, risks and burdens of the treatment in the particular case should be assessed. [Section 17.10]

21. Although ultimately the responsibility for treatment decisions rests with the clinician in charge of the patient's care, it is important, where non-emergency decisions are made, that account is taken of the views of other health professionals involved in the patient's care and people close to the patient, in order to ensure that the decision is as well informed as possible. In Scotland, certain other people will have a legal right to be consulted under the Adults with Incapacity (Scotland) Act. [Sections 13.4 and 18.2]

22. Even where their views have no legal status in terms of actual decision making, those close to the patient may have a right to be consulted. In any event it is clear that they can provide important information to help ascertain whether the patient would have considered life-prolonging treatment to be beneficial. [Section 18.3]

23. Good communication, both within the health care team and between the health team and the patient and/or those close to the patient, is an essential part of decision making. Wherever possible, consensus should be sought amongst all those consulted about whether the provision of life-prolonging treatment would benefit the patient. [Section 18.4]

24. Decisions to withhold or withdraw conventional treatment, on the basis that it is not providing a benefit to the patient, should be made by the clinician in overall charge of the patient's care following discussion with the rest of the health care team and, where appropriate, those close to the patient and any appointed health care proxy. Where the clinician's

view is seriously challenged and agreement cannot be reached by other means, review by a court would be advisable. [Section 19.3]

Decisions about withholding or withdrawing artificial nutrition and hydration

25. In England, Wales and Northern Ireland, proposals to withdraw artificial nutrition and hydration from a patient who is in persistent vegetative state, or in a state of very low awareness closely resembling pvs, currently require legal review. [Section 21.1]

26. In Scotland the withdrawal of artificial nutrition and hydration from a patient in pvs does not require a court declaration. [Section 21.2]

27. The courts have not specified that declarations should be sought before withholding or withdrawing artificial nutrition and hydration from patients who are not in persistent vegetative state. Although a body of medical opinion has developed that such action would be appropriate in some cases (such as some patients who have suffered a serious stroke or have severe dementia), United Kingdom courts have not yet considered such a case. This arguably leaves doctors in an area of legal uncertainty and therefore open to challenge particularly following implementation of the Human Rights Act. [Sections 19.3 and 21.4]

28. The BMA believes that the following additional safeguards should be applied to decisions to withhold or withdraw artificial nutrition and hydration from patients whose death is not imminent and whose wishes are not known. [Section 22.1]

    (a) All proposals to withhold or withdraw artificial nutrition and hydration whether in hospital or in the community should be subject to formal clinical review by a senior clinician who has experience of the condition from which the patient is suffering and who is not part of the treating team.

    (b) In England, Wales and Northern Ireland, where it is proposed to withdraw artificial nutrition and hydration from a patient in persistent vegetative state or a state closely resembling pvs, legal advice should be sought and a court declaration is likely to be required until such time as the courts have stated otherwise. (It is also advisable for medical teams facing the same situation in Scotland to consider carefully whether similar recourse to the courts should not also be initiated.)

(c) All cases in which artificial nutrition and hydration has been withdrawn should be available for clinical review to ensure that appropriate procedures and guidelines were followed. Anonymised information should also be available to the Secretary of State on request and, where applicable, the Commission for Health Improvement.

PART 4 – Once a decision has been reached to withhold or withdraw life-prolonging treatment

29. The basis for the decision to withhold or withdraw life-prolonging treatment should be carefully documented in the patient's medical notes. [Section 25.1]

30. Decisions to withhold or withdraw life-prolonging treatment should be reviewed before and after implementation to take account of any change in circumstances. [Section 25.2]

31. Decisions to withdraw or withhold life-prolonging treatment should be subject to review and audit. [Section 25.3]

32. Although not responsible for making the decision to withhold or withdraw treatment, those close to the patient are often left with feelings of guilt and anxiety in addition to their bereavement. It is important that the family is supported both before and after the decision has been made to withdraw or withhold life-prolonging treatment. [Section 26.1]

33. The emotional and psychological burden on staff involved with withdrawing and withholding life-prolonging treatment should be recognised and adequate support mechanisms need to be available and easily accessible before, during and after decisions have been made. [Section 26.2]

Appendix 1 Some useful addresses

British Association for Parenteral and Enteral Nutrition (BAPEN), PO Box 922, Maidenhead, Berks SL6 4SH

British Medical Association, BMA House, Tavistock Square, London WC1H 9JP. Tel: 020 7387 4499, Fax: 020 7383 6400, Website: http://www.bma.org.uk

Council for Professions Supplementary to Medicine, Park House, 184 Kennington Park Road, London SE11 4BU. Tel: 020 7582 0866, Fax: 020 7820 9684, Website: http://www.cpsm.org.uk

Department of Health, Wellington House, 133-155 Waterloo Road, London SE1 8UG. Tel: 020 7972 2000, Website: http://www.open.gov.uk/doh/dhhome.htm

General Medical Council, 178 Great Portland Street, London W1W 5JE. Tel: 020 7580 7642, Fax: 020 7915 3641, Website: http://www.gmc-uk.org

Law Commission, Conquest House, 37-38 John Street, London WC1N 2BQ. Tel: 020 7453 1220, Fax: 020 7453 1297, Website: http://www.lawcom.gov.uk/lawcomm/

Law Society, 113 Chancery Lane, London WC2A 1PL. DX 56 London/Chancery Lane. Tel: 020 7242 1222, Fax: 020 7831 0344, Website: http://www.lawsociety.org.uk

Law Society of Scotland, 26 Drumsheugh Gardens, Edinburgh EH3 7YR. DX ED1. Tel: 0131 226 7411, Fax: 0131 225 2934, Website: http://www.lawscot.org.uk

Lord Chancellor's Department, Selborne House, 54-60 Victoria Street, London SW1E 6QW. Tel: 020 7210 8500, Website: http://www.open.gov.uk/lcd/lcdhome.htm

Medical Defence Union, 230 Blackfriars Road, London SE1 8PJ. Tel: 020 7202 1500, Fax: 020 7202 1666, Website: http://www.the-mdu.com

Medical and Dental Defence Union of Scotland, Mackintosh House, 120 Blythswood Street, Glasgow G2 4EA. Tel: 0141 221 5858, Fax: 0141 228 1208, Website: http://www.mddus.com

Medical Protection Society, 33 Cavendish Square, London W1G 0PS. Tel: 020 7399 1300, Fax: 020 7399 1301, Website: http://www.mps.org.uk/medical/

Mental Welfare Commission for Scotland, K floor, Argyle House, 3 Lady Lawson Street, Edinburgh EH3 9SH. Tel: 0131 222 6111, Fax: 0131 222 6112, Website: http://www.mwcscot.org.uk

Official Solicitor of the Supreme Court, 81 Chancery Lane, London WC2A 1DD. DX 0012 London/Chancery Lane. Tel: 020 7911 7127, Fax: 020 7911 7105, Website: http://www.offsol.demon.co.uk

Official Solicitor of the Supreme Court for Northern Ireland, Royal courts of Justice, PO Box 410, Belfast BT1 3JF. Tel: 028 9023 5111, Fax: 028 9031 3793

Patients Association, PO Box 935, Harrow, Middlesex HA1 3YJ. Tel: 020 8423 9111, Fax: 020 8423 9119, Website: http://www.pat-assoc.org/

Royal College of General Practitioners, 14 Prince's Gate, Hyde Park, London SW7 1PU. Tel: 020 7581 3232, Fax: 020 7225 3047, Website: http://www.rcgp.org.uk

Royal College of Nursing, 20 Cavendish Square, London W1M 0AB. Tel: 020 7409 3333, Fax: 020 7647 3435, Website: http://www.rcn.org.uk

Royal College of Paediatrics and Child Health, 50 Hallam Street, London W1N 6DE. Tel: 020 7307 5600, Fax: 020 7307 5601, Website: http://www.rcpch.ac.uk

Royal College of Physicians, 11 St Andrew's Place, London NW1 4LE. Tel: 020 7935 1174, Fax: 020 7487 5218, Website: http://www.rcplondon.ac.uk

Royal College of Physicians and Surgeons of Glasgow, 232-242 St Vincent Street, Glasgow G2 5RJ. Tel: 0141 221 6072, Fax: 0141 221 1804, Website: http://www.rcpsglasg.ac.uk

Royal College of Physicians of Edinburgh, 9 Queen Street, Edinburgh EH2 1JQ. Tel: 0131 225 7324, Fax: 0131 220 3939, Website: http://www.rcpe.ac.uk

Royal College of Surgeons of Edinburgh, Nicolson Street, Edinburgh EH8 9DW. Tel: 0131 527 1600, Fax: 0131 557 6406, Website: http://www.rcsed.ac.uk

Royal College of Surgeons of England, 35-43 Lincoln's Inn Fields, London WC2A 3PN. Tel: 020 7405 3474, Fax: 020 7831 9438, Website: http://www.rcseng.ac.uk

Scottish Law Commission, 140 Causewayside, Edinburgh EH9 1PR. Tel: 0131 668 2131, Fax: 0131 662 4900, Website: http://www.scotlawcom.gov.uk

Scottish Office Solicitors, Division C3, Health and Social Work Services, Victoria Quay, Edinburgh EH6 6QQ. Tel: 0131 556 8400

United Kingdom Central Council for Nursing, Midwifery and Health Visiting (UKCC), 23 Portland Place, London W1N 4JT. Tel: 020 7637 7181, Fax: 020 7436 2924, Website: http://www.ukcc.org.uk

Notes and References

1. For example, guidance on clinical aspects of the diagnosis of persistent vegetative state is provided by the Royal College of Physicians (RCP), guidance on artificial nutrition and hydration is provided by the British Association of Parenteral and Enteral Nutrition (BAPEN) and guidance on treatment decisions for children is issued by the Royal College of Paediatrics and Child Health (RCPCH).
2. This guidance covers the legal situation in England, Wales, Scotland and Northern Ireland. Those working elsewhere need to take account of the law in the relevant jurisdiction. Also it has to be recognised that the Human Rights Act is a very new and revolutionary measure, and how exactly it is to be interpreted remains to be seen.
3. *Airedale NHS Trust v Bland* [1993] 1 All ER 821.
4. *Re R (Adult: Medical Treatment)* [1996] 2 FLR 99.
5. *Re J (A Minor) (Wardship: Medical Treatment)* [1990] 3 All ER 930.
6. For more specific guidance on the provision and withdrawal of artificial nutrition and hydration see: British Association for Parenteral and Enteral Nutrition (BAPEN). *Ethical & Legal Aspects of Clinical Hydration and Nutritional Support*. London: BAPEN, 1998. Also, British Geriatrics Society and Royal College of Nursing. *Guidelines on Artificial Hydration and Nutrition in Elderly Patients*. London: BGS/RCN, 1997.
7. *Airedale NHS Trust v Bland* [1993], op cit.
8. See, for example, *Frenchay Healthcare NHS Trust v S* [1994] 1 WLR 601, *Re D (Medical Treatment)* [1998] 1 FLR 411 and *Law Hospital NHS Trust v Lord Advocate* (1996) SLT 848.
9. Treloar A, Howard P. Tube Feeding: Medical Treatment or Basic Care? *Catholic Medical Quarterly* 1998; August: 5-7.
10. The Law Commission. *Report No 231 Mental Incapacity*. London: Law Commission, 1995: 90-93.
11. Baines MJ. Symptom management and palliative care. In: Evans JG, Williams TF, editors. *Oxford Textbook of Geriatric Medicine*. Oxford: OUP, 1992: 693-6.
12. *Airedale NHS Trust v Bland* [1993], op cit.
13. Human Rights Act 1998 s6(6).
14. This was the example used in *Re MB (Medical Treatment)* [1997] 2 FLR No 3.
15. *St George's Healthcare National Health Service Trust v S* (No 2): *R v Louize Collins & Ors, Ex Parte S* (No 2) [1998] 3 WLR 936. See also, Department of Health. *Consent to Treatment – Summary of Legal Rulings*. 1999, HSC 1999/031.

16. *Paton v UK* (1980) 19 DR 244, 3 EHHR 408.
17. These arguments are set out in some detail in British Medical Association. *Advance Statements About Medical Treatment.* London: BMA, 1995. See also, The Patients Association. *Advance Statements About Future Medical Treatment: A Guide for Patients.* London: The Patients Association, 1996.
18. *Re C (Adult: Refusal of Treatment)* [1994] 1 WLR 290.
19. This issue was discussed in a consultation paper from the Lord Chancellor's Department in 1997 entitled: *Who Decides? Making Decisions on Behalf of Mentally Incapacitated Adults.* In 1999, however, the Government announced its legislative plans for decision making on behalf of incapacitated adults in its report *Making Decisions: The Government's Proposals for Making Decisions on Behalf of Mentally Incapacitated Adults.* Advance directives are not part of these plans and the Government made clear that, for the time being, the common law and the BMA code of practice provided a sufficiently clear and flexible framework.
20. See, for example, *Airedale NHS Trust v Bland* [1993], op cit, *Re T (Adult: Refusal of Treatment)* [1993] Fam 95 and *Re C (Adult: Refusal of Medical Treatment)* [1994], op cit.
21. British Medical Association. *Advance Statements About Medical Treatment*, op cit.
22. See, for example, *Re J (A Minor) (Child in Care: Medical Treatment)* [1992] 3 WLR 507.
23. See *R V. North West Lanashire Health Authority, ex parte A, D & G* [2000] 1 WLR 977.
24. British Medical Association and The Law Society. *Assessment of Mental Capacity: Guidance for Doctors and Lawyers.* London: BMA, 1995.
25. Mental Health Act 1983. Mental Health (Scotland) Act 1984.
26. *Re MB (Medical Treatment)* [1997], op cit.
27. This is one of the recommendations made in The Lord Chancellor's Department's Green Paper: *Who Decides? Making Decisions on Behalf of Mentally Incapacitated Adults*, December 1997.
28. *Re F (Mental Patient: Sterilisation)* [1990] 2 AC 1.
29. Adults with Incapacity (Scotland) Act 2000. Part 5 deals with medical treatment and research. The Scottish Executive has stated that implementation of the Adults with Incapacity (Scotland) Act 2000 will commence in April 2001 and be completed in April 2002. Additional regulations and codes of practice to implement the Act will also be issued.
30. Nelson L J *et al.* Forgoing Medically Provided Nutrition and Hydration in Pediatric Patients. *Journal of Law, Medicine & Ethics* 1995; **23**:33-46.
31. The Royal College of Paediatrics and Child Health has published its views of a framework for decision making which identifies ethical issues which arise in decisions to withdraw or withhold treatment. Royal College of Paediatrics and Child Health. *Withholding or*

Withdrawing Life Saving Treatment in Children. London: RCPCH, 1997.

32. *Re J (A Minor) (Wardship: Medical Treatment)* [1990], op cit.
33. Children Act 1989 s1(3). Similar provisions are made in the Children (Scotland) Act 1995 s11(7) and The Children (Northern Ireland) Order 1995 art 3(1).
34. Not all parents have parental responsibility. Both parents have parental responsibility if they were married at the time of the child's conception, or birth, or at some time after the child's birth. Neither parent loses parental responsibility if they divorce. If the parents have never married, only the mother automatically has parental responsibility. The father may acquire it by entering into a parental responsibility agreement with the mother and registering it in the Principal Registry of the Family Division of the High Court, or through a parental responsibility order made by a court.

    The Government has announced its intention to amend these rules, following a consultation exercise carried out in 1998 by the Lord Chancellor's Department, so that parental responsibility is automatically conferred on unmarried fathers who sign the child's birth certificate along with the mother. This requires a change in legislation and, at the time of writing, it has not been established when these changes will take place.

    Parents who do not have parental responsibility lack the legal authority to give consent but play an essential role in determining best interests and in the decision making process and may be entitled to participate under the Human Rights Act.
35. British Medical Association. *Medical Ethics Today: Its Practice and Philosophy.* London: BMA, 1993: 76.
36. *Re C (Medical Treatment)* [1998] 1 FLR 384.
37. *A National Health Service Trust v D & Ors* (2000) TLR 19 July 2000.
38. *Re T (A Minor) (Wardship: Medical Treatment);* sub nom *Re C (A Minor) (Parents' Consent to Surgery)* [1997] 1 All ER 906.
39. *Gillick v Wisbech Area Health Authority* [1986] AC 122. Age of Legal Capacity (Scotland) Act 1991 s2(4).
40. In Scotland the law provides that from the age of 12 a child should be presumed to be of sufficient age and maturity to form a view, Children (Scotland) Act 1995 s16(2).
41. Alderson P, Montgomery J. *Health Care Choices: Making Decisions with Children.* London: Institute for Public Policy Research, 1996.
42. Ondrusek N, Abramovitch R, Pencharz P, Koren G. Empirical Examination of the Ability of Children to Consent to Clinical Research, *Journal of Medical Ethics* 1998; **24**(3):158-65.
43. British Medical Association. *Consent, Rights and Choices in Health Care for Children and Young People.* London: BMJ Books, 2001. Chapter 5 discusses competence and its assessment.
44. Family Law Reform Act 1969 s 8 and Age of Majority Act (NI) 1969 art 4.
45. *Gillick v Wisbech Area Health Authority* [1986], op cit.

46. Ibid.
47. *Re R (A Minor)* [1991] 4 All ER 177.
48. *Re W (A Minor) (Medical Treatment)* [1992] 4 All ER 649.
49. Elliston S. If you Know What's Good for You: Refusal of Consent to Medical Treatment by Children. In: McLean SAM, editor. *Contemporary Issues in Law, Medicine and Ethics.* Aldershot: Dartmouth, 1996.
50. British Medical Association. *Medical Ethics Today: Its Practice and Philosophy,* op cit:85.
51. Age of Legal Capacity (Scotland) Act 1991.
52. Children Act 1989 s 1(3). Children (Scotland) Act 1991 s 6(1), s 16(2). UN Convention on the Rights of the Child 1989 (Article 12). See also Human Rights Act 1998, s 1 and Schedule 1, Articles 8 and 10.
53. The Royal College of Nursing. *Restraining, Holding Still and Containing Children: Guidance for Good Practice.* London: RCN, 1999.
54. Guidance is available from a variety of sources about treatment decisions for patients in persistent vegetative state. See, for example, Royal College of Physicians. The Permanent Vegetative State. *Journal of the Royal College of Physicians* 1996; **30**:119-121. See also, British Medical Association. *BMA Guidelines on Treatment Decisions for Patients in Persistent Vegetative State.* London: BMA, June 1996 And also, The Multi-Society Task Force on PVS. Medical Aspects of the Persistent Vegetative State (Part Two). *New England Journal of Medicine* 1994; **330**:1572-79.
55. See, for example, British Medical Association, Resuscitation Council (UK) and Royal College of Nursing. *Decisions Relating to Cardiopulmonary Resuscitation.* London: BMA, 1999.
56. See, for example, Secker AB, Meier DA, Mulvihill MPH, Paris BEC. Substituted Judgment: How Accurate Are Proxy Predictions? *Annals of Internal Medicine* 1991; **115**(2):92-8. See also, Gerety MB, Chiodo LK, Kanten DN, Tuley MR, Cornell JE. Medical Treatment Preferences of Nursing Home Residents: Relationship to Function and Concordance with Surrogate Decision-Makers. *Journal of the American Geriatrics Society* 1993; **41**:953-960. And also, Emanuel EJ, Emanuel LL. Proxy Decision Making for Incompetent Patients: An Ethical and Empirical Analysis. *Journal of the American Medical Association* 1992; **267**:2067-2071.
57. The right to respect for privacy under Article 8 is not an absolute right.
58. *R v Woollin* [1998] 4 All ER 103.
59. *NHS Trust A v Mrs M; NHS Trust B v Mrs H* [2000] TLR 29/11/2000.
60. This resolution was passed at the BMA's Annual Representative Meeting in 1997.
61. *Re F (Mental Patient: Sterilisation)* [1990], op cit.
62. *Re R (Adult: Medical Treatment)* [1996], op cit.
63. *Re J (A Minor) (Child in Care: Medical Treatment)* [1992], op cit.

64. *Law Hospital NHS Trust v Lord Advocate*, (1996), op cit.
65. See, for example, Lennard-Jones JE. Giving or Withholding Fluids and Nutrients: Ethical and Legal Aspects. *Journal of the Royal College of Physicians of London* 1999; **33**(1):39-45.
66. Up to date information may be obtained from the BMA's website or by contacting the Medical Ethics Department at the British Medical Association.

Index